Disability

24 JUN 2022

AWN

Disability: Controversial debates and psychosocial perspectives examines a range of theories and practices in relation to disability. The focus of the work is not disabled people as 'objects' of study, but rather an analysis of disability as it has been historically and culturally constructed, and psychically experienced.

The book shows that the analysis of disability raises key questions about the organisation of difference within a range of relationships, practices and institutions, around the categories of 'intellect', 'functional capacity', 'normality' and 'beauty'.

The chapters cover:

- values and ethics
- medicine and allied professions
- the social construction of disability
- causes and process of categorising 'impairment'
- unconscious investments and interpersonal relationships
- disabling images.

Disability is a major issue that our society faces and, with controversial debates over the provision of benefits and services, this book will be essential reading for students of social work, cultural studies, disability studies, counselling and psychotherapy and social policy.

Deborah Marks is course director of the MA in Disability Studies at the Centre for Psychotherapeutic Studies, University of Sheffield.

D0281722

UNIVERSITY OF LONDON
INSTITUTE OF EDUCATION
LIBRARY

Disability

Controversial debates and
psychosocial perspectives

Deborah Marks

COLLEGE OF RIPON
AND YORK ST JOHN
LIBRARY

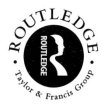

London and New York

First published 1999
by Routledge
11 New Fetter Lane, London EC4P 4EE

Simultaneously published in the USA and Canada
by Routledge
29 West 35th Street, New York, NY 10001

Routledge is an imprint of the Taylor & Francis group

© 1999 Deborah Marks

Typeset in Times by Routledge
Printed and bound in Great Britain by Biddles Ltd,
Guildford and King's Lynn

All rights reserved. No part of this book may be reprinted or
reproduced or utilised in any form or by any electronic,
mechanical, or other means, now known or hereafter
invented, including photocopying and recording, or in any
information storage or retrieval system, without permission in
writing from the publishers.

British Library Cataloguing in Publication Data
A catalogue record for this book is available from the British
Library

Library of Congress Cataloging in Publication Data
Disability: controversial debates and psychosocial
perspectives/Deborah Marks
Includes bibliographical references and index.
1. Disability studies. 2. Sociology of disability
3. Handicapped. I. Title.
HV1568.2.M37   1999
362.4–dc21   99-14620
CIP

ISBN 0–415–16202–5 (hbk)
ISBN 0–415–16203–3 (pbk)

To Gaby and Maurice

Contents

Preface

There is something about being told that you're at least as good as
everyone else. If you hear it often enough you begin to doubt it.
(LaRossa, quoted in Sivanandan, 1985: 243)

What is disability? Where might we find it? These might sound like
silly questions. The common-sense answer which most people give is
that a disability is what someone has 'when their body or mind
doesn't work properly'. For example, a person who is 'paralysed or
brain-damaged' is disabled. In popular imagery disability continues
to be perceived as being about specific impairments (such as blindness and paralysis) or forms of assistance and technologies (such as
guide-dogs and wheelchairs). Such a 'model' of disability assumes
that disability is a tragic aberration which afflicts a minority of
people. This common-sense assumption is pervasive. It shapes much
of the medical, social and educational treatment of disabled people.
It also shapes the structure of our environments – for example the
way transport systems, buildings and institutions are built and
organised.

Disability Studies is a field for debate and critique of these
'common-sense' notions and the way in which disability is understood, treated and experienced. It challenges the reductive focus on
an 'essential' disabled person in favour of an exploration of the
ways in which people are socially constructed within the context of
a range of disabling environments. This book reviews and critically
engages with these debates. I argue that it is important to develop a
dynamic understanding of disability, which recognises the importance of examining the interrelationship between embodied
subjects, and complex social and psychic relationships. I examine

aspects of bodily and psychic experience, and their relevance in thinking about the substantial body of critical cultural and socio-logical work already undertaken within Disability Studies. As such, this book challenges some of the Cartesian dualities around the mind/body and individual/society, which shape assumptions about disability.

Disability is a major issue faced by our society. Debates over the provision of benefits and services, legislation preventing discrimina-tion and questions of how to foster social inclusion present some of the most pressing contemporary policy concerns and issues. They raise questions not just about the treatment but also about the defi-nition of disability. Disability Studies has made an important contribution in generating new critical thinking.

Disability Studies emerged as an academic discipline out of the pioneering work of disabled scholars and activists, who found that disability, as a socially constructed phenomenon, was not being critically addressed within the traditional academic disciplines. As such, there was a need for a new, cross-disciplinary approach, which drew upon different levels of analysis, from the macro to the micro, within sociology, political science, the humanities (literature and film studies, human geography), philosophy, psychology, the arts, architecture and design. As the burgeoning field of Disability Studies develops, important attempts have been made to open dialogue with traditional academic disciplines, such as the recent fruitful debate between medical sociology and Disability Studies (Barnes and Mercer, 1996). Other debates, about the relative impor-tance of the humanities and culture compared to policy and politics, have been the source of much discussion between researchers from the UK and USA (in the 'Disability Research' email discussion group). Such dialogue and cross-fertilisation of ideas continues to be a central characteristic of Disability Studies.

However, a recent trend towards demarcating the 'proper' range of Disability Studies indicates an opposing insular tendency to define certain approaches as outside the boundaries of the discipline. In particular, some scholars have argued that Disability Studies has an emancipatory agenda that is incompatible with rehabilitation, medical or psychological approaches. Linton (1998), for example, argues that approaches with a 'remedial' endeavour, such as program-mes concerned with the training of health care workers cannot be considered to be Disability Studies because they lack the critical social, political and cultural perspective.

In this book, I wish to challenge what I consider to be a narrowing of the discipline's focus towards a purely social perspective and I aim to introduce one theoretical approach that has been absent from debates so far, and this is psychoanalysis. Subjective and unconscious investments, identifications and the management of differences play a crucial role in the construction and experience of disability. However, because of the way psychology has, in the past, pathologised disabled people (Oliver, 1990; Lenny, 1994), it has not been seen as useful or relevant to critical discussion within Disability Studies. I argue that it is important to differentiate mainstream psychology, with its individualising cognitive, behavioural and social schools, from some of the more radical and critical strands of psychoanalytic thought.

Whilst the field is still relatively young, it is becoming an increasingly important feature on the academic landscape. Until recently Disability Studies had not established the paraphernalia which accompany an established research area. Now there are two academic journals devoted to the critical study of disability from a social perspective (*Disability and Society* and *Disability Studies Quarterly*) and a growing number of textbooks and readers (Swain *et al.*, 1994; Hales, 1996; Davis, 1997; Shakespeare, 1998). The creation of disciplines such as Women's Studies and African-American Studies offer an important space for critical work and serve as precursors to the inclusion of critical reflections on disability as a key feature of mainstream academic exploration.

Mike Oliver (1991) wrote of his edited book on *Social Work* that 'this book is aimed at a moving target' because the world of social work has been placed under continual scrutiny. The same could surely be said of critical thinking about disability. There are many heated debates in the field, over questions both of theory and practice, that mark a very exciting period of intellectual ferment. This book aims to explore some of these conflicts.

Positioning the author

In the early stages of writing this book I had a dream. I was cycling up a staircase alongside a colleague who used a wheelchair. He was climbing the stairs using an electric wheelchair which had caterpillar wheels. He had no difficulty negotiating the terrain. I was completely exhausted and found it increasingly difficult to sustain the pace at which my colleague was travelling. Eventually I could go no further.

Drenched in sweat and shaking all over, I began to slide down the hill. My colleague finally grabbed a rope, and with a patient sigh, attached it to my bike and pulled me up the stairs.

The dream offers a vivid demonstration of the social model of disability, which looks at the way people are disabled by the social and environmental context. It reverses traditional assumptions about who has 'the problem' since it is the non-disabled cyclist who needs assistance from the disabled wheelchair user. Such a reversal helps to deconstruct the fixed opposition between disability and ability. It also examines the interpersonal dynamics which govern a situation in which assistance is required. I am made to feel ashamed by my need for assistance from my able (disabled) colleague.

On a more personal level, my dream about cycling up the stairs with my colleague seems to express anxiety about my position as a non-disabled person entering a discipline and terrain pioneered by disabled people. Many of us would be suspicious of a white woman teaching anti-racism. So there are clearly issues around the way in which I theorised my position. As well as the whole question of material interests which will be a central concern of this book, it is also important to examine emotional investments. In addition to the conscious reasons which make the study of disability so compelling for any critical researcher, my dream raises questions about my unconscious motivation for engaging with the topic of disability. It is important, if I am advocating an analysis of emotional experience, to reflect upon my own in relation to disability. This concern would be dismissed by many traditional researchers as irrelevant and unscientific. It takes us away from the subject we are studying. Other more politically progressive or radical scholars see such self-reflection as individualistic. Feminist researchers, by contrast, have, for the last two decades, been concerned to reflect upon the location and investments of the writer or researcher in relation to her work. In part, speculation about my personal investments in this book became necessary because my position as a non-disabled woman running a course in Disability Studies calls forth the spectre of colonisation of the 'Other', which has been spoken about by many writers on feminism, disability, racism and heterosexism (Marks, 1996a; Wilkinson and Kitzinger, 1996).

I want to address my own sense of identity and difference in relation to disability in order to address the dilemmas engendered by my position as member of a privileged group of 'able-bodied' people. I hope this will show that the question of psychological as well as social motivation is central to our understanding of the relationship between non-disabled and disabled people. It behoves all people working around issues of oppression to acknowledge their own structural location, even if this location is not seen as being immutable, but is rather performed to reflect upon, although not necessarily make publicly available, their own personal motives. Failure to reflect on what the member of the privileged group is getting out of the encounter may serve to mystify their position. This is why it is important to locate oneself and one's investments in the analysis. Recognising and validating difference, and also acknowledging points of identity remain central features of the psychoanalytic enterprise.

My own interest in disability began with work in the field of mental illness and learning difficulty, both in terms of voluntary and academic work. I have since realised that these two areas represented issues which so many of us struggle with, around the feeling and fear of being mad, alien and stupid, and also the guilt about having avoided being publicly placed within these categories of people. One way in which many academics and people working in the caring professions deal with their (possibly unconscious) emotional burdens is to attend to them vicariously, through the study or care of others. As Skynner puts it in relation to those choosing to work in the 'caring' professions, 'discouraged from direct study of ourselves, we can nevertheless gratify our curiosity at one remove, by studying others and helping them to grow instead' (1991: 196). However, this leads to the somewhat dangerous investment which such people have in those they see as the 'ones with the problem', and to failing to appreciate the way environments disable people. By disavowing all ownership of difficulty and projecting it onto others, it becomes difficult to allow the 'mad' and 'stupid' people to become sane and intelligent. As such, it has been important for my own development to own difficulties and to acknowledge identifications as well as differences I had with the people I worked with and tried to understand.

My move from the fields of learning and emotional difficulties (which remain the key areas of my research) into the wider area of 'Disability Studies' came initially, through reading the work of Mike Oliver and realising that his work on barriers offered a far more radical, important and thorough-going challenge to individualistic and pathologising conceptions of disability. His work offered a way of linking a range of oppressions and seeing the value of a cross-disability perspective. This book is an attempt to link a cross-disability barriers-centred approach with a grounded, contextualised, culturally specific exploration of differences. Learning about the social model of disability has, like being introduced to Marxism and psychoanalysis, changed everything.

Acknowledgements

My biggest debt of gratitude goes to Valerie Sinason whose pioneering clinical work and writing has taught me so much. Attending the Mental Handicap Workshop at the Tavistock was an enormous privilege and a profound learning experience. I am also deeply grateful to Brett Khar for giving me generous encouragement and advice.

Next I wish to acknowledge all the academics and activists who have made such a crucial contribution to the MA course at Sheffield in Disability Studies, and especially to Mike Oliver. Thank you to colleagues at the Centre for Psychotherapeutic Studies, and especially to Bob Young for offering such engaged disagreement. I also wish to acknowledge the contribution to my thinking made by the thoughtful, critical and passionate students who have taken the MA Disability Studies at Sheffield. I wish I had the space to mention past and present students by name.

Erica Burman, Martin Miller, Ian Parker, Paul Reizin and David Ward have been very important in the process of writing this book. Gaby Marks, Adah Sachs and Sue Vice read sections and offered excellent comments. Jessica Evans and the Science Museum supplied slides. Finally, and most importantly, I am indebted to Maurice Marks for being a stalwart of support and, as always, for helping me to see the wood for the trees, and to Dan Marks for detailed, thorough and much needed critical editing.

Introduction

This book argues that the analysis of disability raises key questions about the organisation of difference within a range of relationships, practices and institutions, around the categories of 'intellect', 'functional capacity', 'normality' and 'beauty'. As such, each chapter takes up a controversy within social theory, and explores its ramifications for ways of seeing disability. Specifically, examination is made of the body, social institutions, cultures, architectural environments, symbolic structures, interpersonal and embodied practices and unconscious experiences. At different points in the book, I identify the value of different theoretical approaches for illuminating a particular question. The approaches I identify as being most useful are as follows: the social model of disability, which focuses on the social and environmental barriers that oppress some impaired people; phenomenology, which addresses interpersonal and experiential aspects of disability; post-structuralism, which focuses on discourses which constitute disability; and psychoanalysis, which addresses intra-psychic experiences of and defences against disability. Conventionally, these theories are seen as mutually incompatible or opposing. However, I argue that they offer complementary and interesting ways of understanding the structures and meanings associated with disability in contemporary British and North American society.

I argue that any study of disability must be grounded within a specific historical context. I begin with an outline of medical values and practices. Then I identify a range of social understandings of disability. In the latter part of the book I move into the discursive realm, identifying a range of representations of disability. Throughout I argue that psychoanalysis brings a new and important embodied and psychological dimension to the critical analysis of disability. Since psychoanalysis has a foot in both medical and social camps, and yet represents an important challenge to both, it offers an important way of bringing about fruitful interdisciplinary dialogue. However, the starting point for any critical understanding must be the notion of civil rights and disabled people's resistance to oppression. This is because it has only been through disabled people's increasing visibility and refusal to accept 'ablist' essentialising binary categories of ability/disability that we come to be in the position of questioning the way disability is produced and treated. Prior to such resistance, disability was seen as a natural misfortune or tragedy. Now that consensus has been disturbed.

Self-representation

Disability rights

In most countries the statutory rights of disabled people to social inclusion lag far behind the rights of other minorities. Whilst we have accepted terms which describe prejudice on the basis of age, race and sex pejoratively (in ageism, racism and sexism), we do not have a widely used name to refer to prejudice on the basis of disability. Terms such as 'disablism' have not yet achieved common currency. Indeed, recent Disability Discrimination Act (1996) in the UK allowed for 'justifiable discrimination' against disabled people, a caveat absent from anti-sexist and anti-racist legislation. Disabled people remain one of the poorest and most oppressed sectors of society in the UK and the USA. Defining the problem of disability as a civil rights matter has been a central goal of a growing number of organisations of disabled people. In 1989 Driedger entitled his book on the disability movement *The Last Civil Rights Movement*. This claim is problematic, since one common feature of oppression is that your struggles are not seen as relevant to the civil rights agenda. For the same reason that many people do not see disability as a civil rights issue, there may be other people who have not come together as a self-identified group to demand greater equity. However, the general suggestion made by Driedger that a strong case may be made to show that disabled people are both socially oppressed and that this oppression was unrecognised, at least until the 1980s, is a powerful one.

A brief historical-geography of the disabled people's movement

Tracing the history of disabled people's struggle for self-representation, respect and citizenship rights has only just begun, with some histories having now been written both about organisations of (rather than for) disabled people (Hasler, 1993) and about the pioneers of the movement (Campbell and Oliver, 1996; Shapiro, 1994).

Disabled people have, since the early 1980s, become an increasingly visible and important lobby. In the USA the disability movement was successful in lobbying the Republican government under George Bush to pass the Americans with Disabilities Act, which extends far-reaching civil rights to disabled people. In the UK, the disabled people's movement has attracted national recognition over a range of dramatic protests organised by groups such as the Disability Action Network. The strength of organisations at the local (e.g. various disabled people's coalitions and fora), national (e.g. the British Council of Disabled People, the umbrella organisation run by and for disabled people and representing 136 organisations), and even international (e.g. the Disabled People's International) levels has done much to challenge the isolation and increase the strength and pride of disabled people.

It is useful to examine the orientation of different theorists in terms of the social and cultural climate in which their ideas were developed, and to contrast the histories of the disability movements in the UK and the USA. The disabled people's movements in Britain and the USA reflect the political culture from which they have emerged. The British movement has been shaped to a greater extent by socialist thought which focuses on the organisation of work as well as the production and distribution of property and ideas. The latter movement has placed greater emphasis on consumer rights and cultural difference.

In the UK scholarship developed out of political protest among physically disabled people. A number of disabled scholars and activists (such as Mike Oliver, Paul Abberley, Vic Finkelstein and Paul Hunt) developed what has come to be known as the 'social model' of disability. This model focused on the social and institutional structures in which certain physical, emotional and intellectual 'differences' are identified and treated. The social model sees disability as the effect of an environment which discriminates against and disables certain 'impaired' individuals. Many early activists came together to form UPIAS, the Union of Physically Impaired People Against Segregation. This radical organisation focused on the material bases of oppression. The social model thus sees the economy as well as state institutions such as the education system and social services as the key factors shaping the oppression of disabled people. Disabled people are united by a shared experience of exclusion and prejudice. There is a strong emphasis among UK pioneers on the importance of resisting the institutional segregation of disabled people.

Social model theorists have been particularly concerned to challenge medical sociology which has been accused of inappropriately equating disability with illness. Many disabled people are not ill and do not need any medical care or treatment. Before disabled scholars entered the field, disability tended to be seen as a problem to be empirically examined by practitioners in applied studies such as health care and social work, rather than as a relational concept which has ramifications for the way in which everyone thinks, feels and acts. Work tended to focus on the question of the 'prevalence and character of chronic illness, and on patient compliance, and ... its associated social problems' (Barnes and Mercer, 1996: 3).

Rather than focusing on the 'impairments' which distinguish disabled people from one another, the social model brings a cross-disability perspective. Instead of examining the particular problems which arise from the negative state of 'not seeing' or 'not being able to walk', the social model looks at the ways in which the environment is designed with a minority of young, fit and non-disabled people in mind.

The Disabled People's Movement in the USA has a markedly different history. Consequently, some British writers have been concerned to distinguish the particular UK history from the North American accounts. John Evans speaks of resistance on the part of UK activists to following the American account of the history of the disability movement.

> I think [there was] a bit of conflict there really of interest and intention and also the pride of being British, of wanting to do our own thing in our own way without these imperialistic Americans telling us what to do. I think in the end what happened was our own version anyway.
>
> (John Evans, quoted in Campbell and Oliver, 1996: 49)

The USA has seen an ever-increasing market for the provision of benefits and services, so that 'people with disabilities' (to use US terminology) have, particularly in the US context, become consumers with an identity and organisation based on their use of services (Albrecht, 1992). The US tradition is also inclined to see disability through the lens of the minority group. Ethnic group membership rather than class has tended to be the central structuring element within US society. The strength and self-confidence of deaf users of American sign language (Padden and Humphries, 1988) has made an important contribution to disability politics in the USA. Second, the politics of experience has been a central tenet of the disabled people's movement in the USA. This is, in part, an effect of the counter-cultural movements of the 1960s, which had a marked influence on a new and assertive group of young men: those returning war veterans who had been disabled whilst serving in Vietnam. Much work has addressed the experience of disability, that is the social psychology or phenomenology of disability, both from the perspective of disabled and non-disabled people (Zola, 1982, 1988; Goffman, 1963). There is a sense of disability needing to be understood not just as a form of economic and structural oppression, but also as a form of exclusion which has been significant in the understanding of identity and self-hood (Wendell, 1996; Davis, 1997; Bogdan; 1988).

It is important, however, not to exaggerate these differences. Disabled scholars and activists in the two countries are equally concerned with campaigns for the removal of disabling environmental barriers, and for the increase of disabled people's autonomy and choice. The focus on architecture has been central to the work of Centres for Independent/Integrated Living and campaigns by ADAPT and DAN over the problem of inaccessible transport. There is a growing disability arts movement in the UK and the USA. There have always been valuable exchanges between disabled people in the two countries. Such cross-fertilisation of ideas and conflict about debates has multiplied in recent years with the growth of Internet discussion groups such as 'Disability Research', which is moderated by Mark Priestley (UK). It currently has about 500 list members and a large contingent of North American members.

Contextually grounded approaches

There is very important critical work on disability emerging from many Western countries such as Sweden and Canada and many non-Western countries. In spite of this, the field of Disability Studies remains dominated by scholars from the UK and the USA. Most anthropological research into disability is based in North America (Ablon, 1984; Edgerton, 1967, Groce, 1985; Murphy, 1987). Despite its universal pretensions, the 'World Institute for Disability' (located in California) carries out research which focuses predominantly on the North American experience. Whilst there is beginning to be some work addressing disability in non-Western cultures (Mallory *et al.*, 1993; Ingstad and Whyte, 1995; Stone, 1996; Miles, 1996), this remains relatively limited. It is important, therefore, to acknowledge the context in which accounts are produced. This book draws primarily upon US and UK traditions. The two countries have such different political traditions and cultures that they offer interesting points of comparison between different experiences and under-standings of disability. It is, however, important to state at the outset that I hope to avoid making universalistic statements which colonise the experiences of those not represented in this text.

This book

In Chapter 1, I examine the question of why an interdisciplinary approach, which attempts to integrate psychic with social perspectives, is so important. I argue that psychoanalytic and post-structuralist conceptions of identity are particularly helpful in thinking critically about the social construction of disability.

In Chapter 2, I look at the whole question of progress. We tend to think of contemporary society as more enlightened and humane regarding the treatment of disabled people than was the case in previous eras. However, I argue that it would be appropriate to adopt a more reflexive and self-critical approach to contemporary values and ethics. This chapter examines the context of what have been identified as cultural death wishes directed at disabled people and actual 'deathmaking'[1] activities practised on disabled people.

In order to develop this critical review of contemporary ethics, Chapter 3 identifies some of the ways in which modern medicine has served to regulate individuals through diagnosing and curing 'pathological states' within them. It identifies a number of iatrogenic (that is medically induced) consequences for the physical and emotional well-being of disabled people.

Chapter 4 outlines those social approaches which locate disability not in damaged bodies but in an oppressive social environment. In this context, the social model of disability offers a crucially important corrective to the hitherto little questioned power of the charities, the disability professions and modern medicine. The chapter also explores some of the criticisms of the social model and subsequent attempts to renew it.

The critical focus on the disabling professions is developed in Chapter 5, which looks at relations both between 'clients' and professionals, and relations among different professional groups. As well as the material interests governing these relationships, I identify some of the psychic investments placed in social constructions of care and need.

In Chapter 6, I focus on the body in an attempt to develop some basic understanding of the causes and nature of impairments. In doing this I attempt to challenge the assumption within some orthodox versions of the social model of disability that impairment has very little relevance to our understanding of disability. I outline structuralist and phenomenological approaches to thinking about embodiment, and discuss the value of including examinations of the experience of different impairments as part of Disability Equality Training.

In Chapter 7, I examine debates about the importance of language in creating and reproducing disability. I reject relativist/idealistic discursive approaches (see Parker, 1998) in favour of a critical realist position which explores some of the psychological investments in certain linguistic constructions.

Chapter 8 continues the discursive debate by examining the importance of visual images in the production and reproduction of disability and, as in the previous chapter, I outline some of the unconscious psychic investments in these images. I suggest that psychoanalysis can serve as a useful ally to a critical epistemology in Disability Studies.

In Closing comments, I return to the question of interdisciplinary work and identify some different ways of resisting disablist oppression and the context within which this resistance takes place.

To summarise, I am concerned to find some way of integrating an understanding of social structures, interpersonal relationships and unconscious motivation in the analysis of disability. Whilst I recognise the value of 'individual' and 'social' models of disability, in order to achieve particular practical and rhetorical ends (e.g. to offer therapy one might wish to focus on an individual, while to challenge a social policy one is likely to focus on environmental barriers), I hope to make the case that as levels of analysis they should not be seen as incompatible.

Interdisciplinary studies, fragmented identities and psychic investments

Disability as a 'specialist' topic

The status of academic knowledge in part reflects the cultural values of society. In the last twenty years, the social study of sexuality has been developing alongside an increasingly confident lesbian and gay liberation movement. Academics from this movement were producing work which for many years was treated as being of marginal interest to mainstream scholarship. Only in the last decade, as the gay liberation movement has become more established, have Lesbian and Gay Studies begun to challenge taken-for-granted assumptions about the nature of heterosexuality (Kitzinger, 1987; Richardson, 1996), rather than the 'problem' of homosexuality.

Disability Studies is a discipline which has grown dramatically in the last ten years yet, unlike Gay and Lesbian Studies, it has still to make a significant mark on social theory. Even those disciplines which deconstruct normalising assumptions regarding the body, the psyche and the intellect, such as post-structuralism and psychoanalysis, rarely employ examples of 'impairment' for the analysis of social processes. Books and journals that purport to deal with 'the body' and 'difference' (e.g. *The Body and Society*) tend rarely to refer to the concept of disability. As Davis puts it, 'the concept of disability has been relegated to a side-show, a freak show at that, far away from the academic midway of progressive ideas and concerns' (Davis, 1995: xi). Davis points out that at academic conferences 'people don't come to sessions on disability. They think it is a specialised area and only the disabled come' (Davis, 1995: xi). Yet the concepts of disability and ability play a central if latent and unacknowledged role in contemporary understandings of normality, the body and intelligence. This book does not examine 'disabled people' but rather explores the construction of disabling experiences and contexts. Its focus is on the way in which people think and feel about, and treat particular kinds of difference.

It is important to consider why the study of disability is seen not as a general issue relevant to all aspects of the human sciences, but rather as a particular and specialised area, relevant only to disabled people. Why, in an intellectual climate of post-structuralism, in which 'realities' such as sex are seen to be socially constructed (Bordo, 1993; Butler, 1993; Gatens, 1993), does disability continue to be treated as if it lies outside the realm of representation or the environment and as if it is firmly located in 'real' damaged bodies or minds? Gerhardt offers one interesting explanation for classical sociology's neglect of physical and mental impairment and illness.

> Sociology may have taken health for granted because Victorian standards of decency held that 'personal' health issues did not deserve the ominous limelight of public attention ... it was shamefully confined to the private quarters of the afflicted person's home and family or neighbourhood. In all, a pervasive distinction prevailed between 'profane' life worlds incorporating matters of physical and mental health, and the 'sacred' world of academic achievement.
>
> (Gerhardt, 1989: xiii)

In other words, sociology, as a relatively young discipline, has been keen to establish academic respectability and thus to mark the 'scientific' study of civil society as its central concern. It wished to avoid those topics associated with private aspects of life. Until the 1970s, sociology was characterised by its marked distinction between the public and the private. Disability, located primarily in the private sphere of the body, was not seen as being relevant to this enterprise, although some of the related policy issues such as welfare provision or public interactions between non-disabled and disabled people were.

It is not surprising that in the universities, which have until recently marked the endpoint of systematic exclusion of disabled people from education, non-disabled people should be unfamiliar with disabled people. Such unfamiliarity has produced an uncomfortable silence around the topic. As in a child told not to stare, the desire to look, combined with the fear of something dangerous and unthinkable, yet intriguing, create a heady mix of prurience, insecurity and avoidance of the subject.

However, it is not enough to examine the difficulties which non-disabled people have in engaging with disability as a social issue. It is also important to explore the underlying social structures which create the category 'disability' in the first place, and the material and emotional investments which maintain the exclusion and oppression of disabled people. Disability should not be conceived as a 'special area' or a topic to be left 'to the experts' (whoever they are conceived to be). Rather, it is a critical resource for social theorising. Nor should disability be treated as an 'add-on' to other forms of social oppression. It is a central and powerful organising principle within contemporary subjectivity and social relations.

Levels of analysis and boundary disputes

The most interesting and useful way to explore disability is not within conventional scholarly boundaries, but rather by drawing upon and challenging the boundaries of mainstream academic disciplines such as psychology and sociology. As such, it is not merely interdisciplinary, but trans-disciplinary (see Curt, 1994): it challenges the validity of the current boundaries and demarcations within the contemporary academic landscape. As with much intellectual inquiry in the 1990s, which focuses on specific topics (such as sexuality, new technologies and environmental politics), this book aims to rethink the aesthetic, ethical, social and relational concepts used by traditional academic disciplines.

There are some writers, such as Turner (1995), who have argued for just such a recognition of the value of theoretical openness to different levels of explanation. As an example, Turner offers a range of ways of interpreting the highly contested 'modern epidemic' of repetitive strain injury (RSI) among those carrying out repetitive tasks in modern office conditions. These include the following. First, since diagnosticians have not been able to identify a clear organic base, some doctors regard RSI as a myth which excuses malingering at work. Second, some commentators identify psychological factors which predispose some workers to suffer from this muscular problem. Third, work conditions (such as the nature of modern equipment) may produce injury. This means that RSI becomes a focal point in political struggles between unions, management and insurance companies. Fourth, RSI is 'a social process by which a "disease" entity was recognised by certain experts' (Turner, 1995: 15). Turner argues that a sociological explanation of RSI (as well as many other chronic conditions) would require the following:

> (1) A phenomenology of pain with a specific inquiry into the sufferer's interpretations and perceptions of the disorder; (2) an analysis of the social processes by which the 'disease' is constituted as a topic by conflicting professional groups with their own vested interest in the existence or disappearance of the problem; and (3) a political economy of the conditions of white-collar employment which, through pressure on the worker, create work processes which produce occupational injuries.
>
> (Turner 1995: 16)

In addition to Turner's sociological explanation, we could also examine RSI as a psycho-somatic condition. A number of psycho-analytic writers, such as McDougal (1974), Broom (1997), and Erskine and Judd (1994) identify some of the complex pathways by which the body can express affects and ideas which have been made inaccessible to conscious awareness.

Turner shows us that we do not necessarily need to see the different accounts as competing because the mind, body and environment are not easily separable entities, but rather mutually constitute each other in complex ways. If one were to use the language of causality, it could be suggested that disability and illness were 'over-determined', that is, they are produced by several factors. We need different levels of analysis to explore different dimensions of experience.

As with any new discipline, what is currently being taught under the rubric of 'Disability Studies' is highly contested. Some approaches to the study of disability focus primarily on 'Disability Awareness Training' or 'Interpersonal Relationships'. Often, the analysis of disability is carried out by those in the 'caring' professions and may form part of professional training. Such work is usually addressed towards the study of a particular 'impairment', such as learning difficulties. The orientation tends to be 'practical' rather than critical and conceptual. Some attempt a more 'scientific' approach, and are rooted in a positivist concern to classify and treat disability through a range of 'preventive' or 'rehabilitative' technologies. Both these approaches tend to adopt current (uncritical) assumptions about what disability is (drawn primarily from an individual/medical model). They focus on disabled people as individuals with damaged bodies (medicine), emotional difficulties (psychology), stigmatised identities (social psychology) and as individuals who represent challenges to public policy (economics, politics and sociology). Within Western culture disabled people symbolise broken, dysfunctional and damaged lives. Within law, geography and architecture, disability has tended to be addressed as a specialised area of work within each field and something which only a minority of people address.

There is very little work which looks at emotional and physical experiences within their social context or the social constitution of psychological and physical experience. This book is ultimately concerned to bring about some dialogue between those working in professions allied to medicine and psychology, and service users and activists. It is also important to foster theoretical dialogue between those attempting to bring about practical changes for excluded groups. Such groups of people may have many fruitful conflicts as well as shared interests. I attempt to bridge the gap between the personal and the political, the internal and the external experiences of disability.

Such an integrative approach is open to criticism from all sides. Social model theorists argue that the focus on impairments is pathologising and oppressive to disabled people. Medical and rehabilitative theories accuse social model theorists of being 'unrealistic' or uncaring about the 'real' problems faced by many disabled people. Finally, psychoanalytic writers accuse social model theorists of a failure to 'come to terms with their problems' and a 'manic denial of loss or difficulty', whilst social model theorists see psychoanalysis as being part of the medical model. I hope to show that the insights brought by different scholarly disciplines need not be seen as mutually exclusive or threatening. I argue that medical, psychological or social models of disability should not be placed in opposition to each other. Each may have ontological and strategic value in deepening a critical understanding of disability.

Ultimately, the study of disability offers a useful topic for deconstructing what Jenks (1998) refers to as 'core sociological dichotomies', for example between structure and agency, continuity and change, fact and value, normal and pathological, culture and nature, public and private, needs and wants, relativism and absolutism.

Identity and subjectivity

The subject in social theory

In addition to demographic, legal and institutional changes in the position of disabled people in Western society, there has been a marked transformation in our understanding of the 'able' body and mind in the late twentieth century. The legacy of feminism and post-structuralism has been to show, in different ways, that intimate relationships are characterised by power relationships and that, to use a well-worn phrase, 'the personal is political'. Further, psycho-analysis, particularly in its institutional and group varieties has shown that the converse is also true: the *political is personal* (Hoggett, 1992; Rustin, 1992; Richards, 1994). That is, what happens in society is shaped by personal investments and unconscious meanings which are invested in and expressed through groups, institutions, cultural and political practices. As such, the last third of the twentieth century within scholarship has seen an increasing problematisation of those theories which make sharp demarcations between individual, group and social spheres (Pringle, 1989).

The discovery (based on the speculations of Silas Weir Mitchell in 1872) that 'phantom limb' phenomena have a neurological basis is currently being used to assist bio-mechanical engineers in the development of 'sophisticated artificial limbs which could actually carry out the "phantom" motions' (Wendell, 1996: 126). Haroway, in her book *Simians, Cyborgs and Women*, argues that since the development of post-Second World War biotechnologies, it has become increasingly difficult to think in terms of 'essential properties'. The once clear distinctions between the categories of human, animal and technological are breaking down in post-modern society. Haroway uses the example of the cyborg to support this case. A cyborg is a hybrid creature, composed of organism and machine or two different kinds of organism. We might see people who use pros-thetic body parts or receive organ donations as cyborgs. However, more significantly, we are all cyborgs to the extent that 'the home, workplace, market, public arena, the body itself can all be dispersed and interfaced in nearly infinite, polymorphous ways. ... The cyborg is a kind of disassembled and reassembled, post-modern collective and personal self' (Haroway, 1991: 163). For example, we can present ourselves in an Internet discussion in any voice we choose. We can reconstruct our face and internal organs and augment parts of our body. We can change sex. Humans may have animal, other human or machine body parts. Debates, for example, about the use of pig hearts in humans, the use of animals to grow human cells that can then be reconnected to human tissue, or the control of computer keyboards through thought rather than muscular contraction have raised not just ethical but also ontological questions (see Figure 1).

How can we distinguish between prosthetics and aids, or even between prosthetics and the 'real' body? Where does the boundary lie between an object which is categorised as part of our body and an object which is seen as an external aid to our body? Many of us would have no problems identifying a pair of spectacles as an aid and a false limb as a prosthetic that replaces or completes a body part. But how, for example, would we categorise a voice augmentation device (which gives the user a 'voice')? Recent disputes about the funding of prosthetics in New York State indicate some of the philosophical difficulties involved. A rehabilitation organisation was engaged in intense lobbying to have voice augmentation devices categorised as 'prosthetics' rather than 'aids'. This is because prosthetics are eligible for (well-resourced) medical funding, since they are seen as replacement body parts, whilst aids are funded by (poorer) social services or individuals' own private means because they are concerned with *assisting* a person rather than becoming *part of* that person. We all have an intuitive sense that a wheelchair or a car is not part of the human body. Yet once we have become familiar with driving or using a wheelchair, we gradually re-evaluate our own bodily boundaries in terms of the technology we are using.

All this suggests that what is initially not 'our body' may become 'our body' in ways that philosophically are indistinguishable from those body parts with which we were born. If the concept of 'wholeness' is thrown into question then the concepts of the broken body and the damaged mind also become philosophically problematic. The post-structuralist work of theorists such as Haroway enables us to challenge the binary distinction between ability and disability. Haroway in her discussion of cyborgs has shown that the boundaries between humanity, machine and animal are becoming increasingly hard to sustain. All the secure essentials which define and differentiate human beings are increasingly held up for questioning.

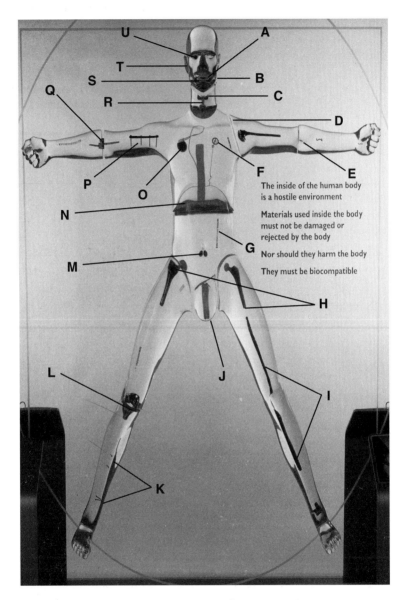

The inside of the human body is a hostile environment

Materials used inside the body must not be damaged or rejected by the body

Nor should they harm the body

They must be biocompatible

Figure 1   Clear Man
Source   Science Museum

Key to diagram
A   Upper dentures: the most common artificial implant?
B   Maxillofacial plate: tiny titanium insert which holds together fractured facial bones while they mend.

C Anterior cervical plate: fuses head and neck bones; prevents excessive movement in a broken neck.

D Shoulder: titanium coated joint, most often given to young arthritis sufferers, such as ex-dancers and professional sportspeople.

E Shape memory alloy bone staples: constructed from a special alloy which contracts when exposed to body heat, so pulling broken bone ends together.

F Artificial heart valve: replaces damaged aortic valve. May be used in conjunction with a pacemaker.

G Sutures: indissoluble 'thread' for stitching wounds.

H Hips: on both right and left, showing the internal and external parts of the joint.

I Distal femoral and tibial nails: quicker to put in than a plate, but not for the squeamish. To insert, simply bang one straight up the centre of the bone.

J Penile prosthesis: bendy, stretchy internal support which helps the recipient maintain an erection.

K External fixation device: pins inserted into the bone support an external 'cage' which will prevent any movement. Used for multiple breaks.

L Knee: another implant commonly found in arthritic ex-dancers and sportspeople.

M Interbody fusion device: used to separate and support vertebrae after diseased discs have been removed.

N Vascular graft: artificial blood vessel. This type is made of polyester.

O Pacemaker: Emits a regular electronic pulse, which artificially stimulates heart contractions.

P Carbon-fibre bone plate: more flexible than metal, so fractures tend to repair themselves with greater speed.

Q Elbow: similar to artificial toe and finger joints.

R Artificial larynx: replaces damaged or diseased vocal cords.

S Dental implant: a titanium 'root', which can be capped.

T Silicone ear: mainly used for cosmetic reconstruction.

U Glass eye: supports the shape of the eyelid when the original eyeball has been damaged.

States, not traits

The social model of disability draws upon a realist philosophical approach which argues that some things (such as impairments) exist independently of the way in which they are socially constructed. There is, at least in principle, an objective, accurate truth, located in an external material reality, which is potentially discoverable. By contrast, post-structuralist theory argues that we can only ever grasp 'versions' of the world. There is no direct perception. The logic of the post-structuralist argument is that not only disability but also impairment is socially constructed.

Post-structuralist theory thus challenges the notion of stable, prior or essential characteristics or identities of people in favour of a much more fluid socially constructed subject. Identities can be seen as sites of enunciation which constitute positions. This raises problems for the disability/ability binary, which places individuals firmly on different sides of an essential divide. I hope to show that the longer we become theoretically absorbed in the question of who is disabled and who is not, the more an answer seems elusive.

One way out of the identity impasse which was adopted by some activists in the late 1980s was to employ the term 'temporarily able bodied' (TAB) to refer to those people who do not identify as disabled. TAB is used with a certain subversive humour, to challenge the security of the 'able-bodied' position. Perhaps a more accurate description of those who do not currently identify as disabled is CAB ('contingently able bodied'[1], which implies the possibility (rather than the inevitability suggested by the term TAB) of future change. CAB has the advantage of more accurately reflecting the precariousness of bodily and mental states. Most people who live beyond 70 years of age will become disabled at some stage in their life. All people are vulnerable to varying levels of serious impairment. Disability is something which many people experience intermittently, for example those with conditions such as ME and MS or those who have a range of chronic diseases which have periods of remission. In addition, most people become disabled, rather than being born disabled, so have experienced the position of being non-disabled. The term CAB thus foregrounds the possibility of disability and the existence of invisible impairments. CAB has the advantage of eschewing the fantasy of 'ability' and the denial of the universality of impairment. Disability is a state that emerges out of a specific constellation of factors. The term 'contingently able bodied' is thus more in tune with contemporary theories of identity and personhood within the social sciences, arts and humanities[2].

Psychic states and structures

The study of disability involves an analysis of the structures and practices which shape our assumptions of the 'normal' and the 'natural'. These socially produced structures are invested with feelings that make attempts to remove disabling barriers seem threatening. Psychic investments in disability have been overlooked in contemporary disability theorising. It is useful to identify some of the similarities between the social model and psychoanalytic accounts in order to justify the usefulness of the latter for our critical theorising. Both show that disablism cannot be removed purely by challenging prejudiced 'attitudes', for example through the provision of 'awareness' training. Structural changes are needed, not just at the legal, economic and political levels, but also at the levels of the organisation of the professions, provision of services, therapeutic practice, and emotional literacy within politics and culture. Both also challenge a narrow medical model which sees the difficulties that many disabled people suffer as being reducible to the effect of their impairments. Finally, both psychoanalysis and Disability Studies resist focus on the unified individual as a unit for analysis or the subject of treatment, in favour of exploration of wider intra- or inter-psychic relationships (as addressed by psychoanalysis) or social systems (as addressed by Disability Studies). The social and psychological relationships represent more than the sum of the individuals that constitute them.

Psychoanalysis, like post-structuralism, has done a great deal to contribute to the erosion of the notion of relatively fixed attitudes and states of mind. Instead of a sharp distinction between the mad and the sane, psychoanalysis shows a continuum of experiences. Just as physical health and impairment exist on a continuum and are not necessarily fixed states, so our mental states are in constant flux, emerging out of a complex constellation of relational, contextual and constitutional factors. Freud offers a model of the psyche which is constructed of conscious and unconscious parts. Ideas which are difficult to integrate into conscious awareness are repressed 'down' into the unconscious, and kept in place by a series of defence mechanisms. Klein's object relations theory[3] identifies processes by which unacceptable ideas are split off from conscious awareness and projected into the world. Anti-psychiatry and systems theory (both of which owe much to psychoanalytic ideas) show that our mental states are not isolated, but rather can only be understood in specific practical settings. The badly behaved or 'disturbed' pupil may be acting as a convenient repository for all the rebellious feelings within a school. We may be expressing a range of emotional states on behalf of other members of a family or an institutional system. In this way, emotional distress, dependency and other 'pathologies' can only be understood in terms of contexts, relationships and meanings. It is important to understand psychic investments in order to make sense of identifications and differences. Psychoanalysis is helpful in examining the mechanisms and contexts in which internalised oppression operates.

I draw upon a particular version of psychoanalytic theory, often referred to as the independent school of British psychoanalysis (see Kohon, 1986; Raynor, 1991; Symington, 1986), which places less emphasis (than classical Freudian and Kleinian approaches) on the role of instincts and more emphasis on the importance of real experiences in the social environment in shaping the psyche. Gomez expresses this view:

> The human being is essentially social; our need for contact with others is primary, and cannot be explained in terms of other needs or reduced to something more basic... our inner world is a changing dynamic process. ... These dynamics influence how we experience external reality and also are themselves influenced by our experience of external reality.
>
> (Gomez, 1997: 1–2)

We can focus on different levels of 'external reality': on interpersonal relationships, for example between the infant and mother; on family dynamics; on wider social fora such as groups (Bion, 1961); on institutions (Menzies Lyth, 1990); or on popular culture (Richards, 1994). As such, the insights of psychoanalysis can be used to look at disability at the socio-cultural, institutional, group and interpersonal levels as well as on the intra-psychic level.

Before looking specifically at some psychic experiences of disability, it will be helpful to outline some of the key psychoanalytic terms used in this book. Whilst there is a risk that attempting to introduce technical terminology will oversimplify complex theories, this risk is out-weighed by the danger of leaving these concepts to the 'clinical experts' and perpetuating the split between socio-cultural and intra-psychic approaches[4].

Defences

When we have thoughts and feelings which cannot be tolerated we defend against them by expelling them from conscious awareness. Bollas (1987) used the term the 'unthought known' to describe experiences which cannot be consciously thought about. They may be experienced as unacceptable for two reasons: either because they conflict with other beliefs and feelings held by the person in question, or because the person finds themselves in an external situation (as much work on trauma has pointed out) that is literally more than they can bear[5]. Examples of the former are when both hatred and concern are felt towards someone who is ill by a person offering assistance, or when a person receiving care feels both resentment and gratitude towards their 'carer'. The wish that the other person 'disappear' is held alongside the value accorded to this person. The less attractive or 'ego-synctonic' sides of a conflict will be the one which is kept unconscious through the deployment of defences. An example of a defence against painful experience is when a newborn baby experiences intense distress if left too long to feel hunger or discomfort, and therefore loses or fails to develop trust in their primary caregivers. Such infants may grow up with difficulties in forming secure attachments to others (Fonagy and Target, 1998). A baby has fewer psychological resources for surviving such experiences because – like a torture victim – it has no idea for how long this state will continue and whether it will get worse (Hurry, 1998). Unmanageably high levels of anxiety lead to the erection of defences which protect a person from painful awareness of conflict or the experience of too much suffering.

Freud's 'talking cure' was concerned to transform 'what is unconscious into what is conscious' (Freud, 1973: 321) and thereby help his patients acknowledge conflicts. The emphasis of much analytic therapy nowadays is less on remembering what has been forgotten than on the ability to 'recognise and accept those parts of the self that have been disowned' (Holmes, 1998: 229). Similarly, an important aspect of this book is the examination of a narcissistic culture in which people strive for 'perfection' and 'independence'. The parts of the self which are unacceptable in a normalising culture (such as bodily imperfection and dependency – we all experience them in varying degrees) are kept outside conscious awareness and come to be split off and projected onto those who have been socially constituted as damaged.

Defences are the various mechanisms or processes which do the work of keeping unbearable conflicts, knowledge and feelings outside conscious awareness. However, defences do not make unconscious ideas and feelings go away. The thoughts and desires continue to exist, although in a 'damned up' or 'strangulated' form (Sandler et al., 1997: 46). Moreover, while serving a protective function, some defences also restrict or distort the actions and thoughts available to a person, thus sabotaging their own goals in life. For example, a person may defend themselves against the pain of rejection and exclusion by taking themselves out of any competitive situation where they might be judged negatively, but in doing so they also lose the opportunity to gain the acceptance which they so desire.

It is helpful to outline some of the ways non-disabled people treat disabled people as 'dustbins of disavowal' (Shakespeare, 1994: 283). Such dynamics explain the complex attraction to and repulsion from disabled people on the part of some non-disabled people. It is hoped that an outline of defences will provide the tools to address the following questions.

- How can we explain the emotional energy (whether of a sadistic, fearful or loving nature) behind so many non-disabled people's responses to the subject of disability?
- How do we explain the patronising, hostile and avoidant ways in which non-disabled people respond to disabled people?
- What is the emotional pay-off which non-disabled people gain from participating in 'altruistic' or 'caring' work, as professionals, support workers or 'carers'?
- What existential anxieties do people habitually repress and how has disability come to represent these feelings?
- Why are disabled people repeatedly constituted in popular culture as dangerous or infantile?

In other words, how might we understand the resistance exhibited by some non-disabled people to the full social inclusion of disabled people? In addition to material interests and social prejudices, what role do subjective identifications and investments play in perpetuating disabling structures. The following section offers a brief outline of some of the key defences which function to keep disabled people isolated and make them available for the 'projections' of non-disabled people.

Splitting

Splitting is a particularly primitive form of defence. There are two forms of splitting. The first refers to the process by which the person doing the splitting avoids ambivalent feelings and endows another person with 'all good' or 'all bad' qualities. This defence can lead to idealisation or denigration of certain people, and prevents recognition of ambivalence and complexity, so that the world is seen in very black and white terms. The second form splitting can take involves projecting unacceptable feelings on to another. Dependency presents a particularly salient example of non-disabled people's projections. We all experience complete dependency as newborns. Those infants who have had basically good experiences of care in early life are protected from awareness of their vulnerability, because their needs are recognised and responded to by a parent or carer. Those infants who experience their dependency in too raw a state, because they have not received empathic recognition or have been subjected to cruelty, are likely to find any reminders of dependency in later life unbearable (Winnicott, 1992a). For this reason, disabled people come to be the recipients of those split-off feelings of dependency which some non-disabled people cannot own.

Projection

'Projection' is a defence first described by Freud and developed by Klein which explains the way in which unwanted feelings or parts of identity or self may be attributed to external objects. The concept of projection offers one key tool for understanding the psychic mechanisms of prejudice against disabled people. In Chapter 8, I identify some of the ways in which existential and developmental fears about monstrosity and stupidity can be projected onto disabled people, who are then experienced as threatening or pitiful and who are avoided because they serve as an uncomfortable reminder to non-disabled people of disavowed aspects of themselves.

Sinason explores the burden of being a recipient of disablist projections:

> The handicapped child and its parents and workers ... carry a double burden. Not only do they have to face public scrutiny of varying kinds, making a simple trip to a local shop the equivalent of running the gauntlet, but they are also burdened by the projections that come the way of other people's responses. ... Being made the recipient of hostile, patronising or demeaning projections is an experience all minorities experience.
>
> (Sinason, 1992: 27)

Reaction formation

Reaction formation involves going to the opposite extreme to obscure or counter unacceptable feelings. Thus, a person may devote themselves to altruistic work in order to counter unconscious guilt.

Freud makes this particular suggestion when he says that expressions of pity might function to disavow unconscious sadism.

> I have no knowledge of having had any craving in my early childhood to help suffering humanity. My innate sadistic disposition was not a very strong one, so that I had no need to develop this one of its derivatives. ... I felt an overpowering need to understand something of the riddles of the world in which we live and perhaps even to contribute to something of their solution[6].
>
> (Freud, 1933: 253)

Another example of reaction formation can be seen when a person attempting to resist a powerful desire to stare looks in the opposite direction when passing a visibly disabled person in the street. Partridge (1990) offers a vivid description of the range of responses he receives as a person who is facially disfigured.

Rationalisation

Rationalisation involves a person justifying their unconscious impulses without being aware of their true source. Rationalisation can be used to blame victims of aggression for their circumstances. The suggestion that wheelchair users might find the back entrance to a building more convenient to use than coming in through the front door may express not just the material self-interest of the owners wishing to avoid the expense of building an accessible entrance, but also serve as a psychic rationalisation for the wish to keep disabled people out of sight and mind.

Defence mechanisms such as the ones listed above are key ways of understanding sexist, racist and disablist prejudices. If we can see discriminatory treatment of disabled people not merely as ignorance, self-interest or indifference, but also as a reflection of unconscious fears and fantasies, then we need to understand what these fears are about. Whilst exploration of the aetiology of defences is beyond the remit of this text, it is important to identify some of the emotional investments behind affects such as altruism and hatred, which play such key functions in shaping non-disabled people's psychic defences.

Internalised oppression

In addition to exploring non-disabled investments, psychoanalytic theory can help us to understand the ways in which disabled people construct, manage, defend against and resist disabling relationships. Denigration and exclusion are the two key forms of psychic oppression suffered by disabled people. John McDermot (1986) describes the social and subsequent psychic isolation experienced by many disabled people as a form of starvation 'wherein the actual handicap became a minor and subsidiary problem in comparison to being cut off from the avenues and possibilities of future experience' (McDermot,1986: 215). Isolation limits not just the educational, vocational and social opportunities afforded to disabled people. It also limits the opportunities for emotional growth. McDermot's view is that the suffering associated with disability is not simply a consequence of impairment (as in the medical model), or the inconvenience and oppression of social barriers (as in the social model). A full picture must take account of how impairment and disability are emotionally experienced.

In other words, we need to explore the ways in which disabled people respond to disabling society and the consequential relationships which are constructed, not just on a macro-political but also on a psychic level. The concept of 'internalised oppression' is helpful in understanding the relationship between psychological difficulties, social exclusion and denigration. Mason (1992) gives an extremely clear and helpful outline of the term.

> Internalised oppression is not the cause of our mistreatment, it is the result of our mistreatment. It would not exist without the real external oppression that forms the social climate in which we exist. Once oppression has been internalised, little force is needed to keep us submissive. We harbour inside ourselves the pain and the memories, the fears and the confusions, the negative self images and the low expectations, turning them into weapons with which to re-injure ourselves, every day of our lives.
>
> (Mason, 1992: 27)

The point made here by Mason is that it is important to examine not just the relationships which people have with others, but also the relationship they have with themselves. The psychic responses to exclusion, marginalisation or rejection include compliance, resistance, anger, withdrawal and despair. It is important to recognise disabled people's active and dynamic internal, as well as external and political responses to oppression. Although Mason does not mention the 'unconscious', it is important to recognise that internalised oppression is most effective when we are unaware it is there. Some experiences are so painful that we repress them from conscious awareness. Yet they continue to affect self-esteem and shape thoughts and actions. Internalised oppression has been left relatively unexplored in disability theorising.

Summary

I have begun this book by identifying some of the ways in which Disability Studies is institutionally segregated from the mainstream academic disciplines. The role of outsider can present a powerful position from which to challenge social and intellectual assumptions about normality and difference. A 'trans-disciplinary' approach, which draws upon theories of the social environment, culture and unconscious experience, not only helps to give a deep and complex picture of the construction and treatment of disability, but also presents a challenge to conventional scholarly boundaries. Whilst the most appropriate starting point is with a materialist account of social institutions and practices, social constructionism and psychoanalysis offer cultural and emotional dimensions to the socio-political framework.

Valuing lives

Introduction

The next two chapters offer a critique of the latent prejudices about disability within contemporary culture and the way these values shape medical treatment and experiences of disability. Whilst some of the material discussed here may be considered inflammatory and one-sided, it is important to identify some of the ways in which medicine has contributed to the oppression of disabled people in order to move on to explore the possibilities for developing a more collaborative dialogue between medical, social and psychological approaches. For this reason, in this chapter, I outline some of the latent assumptions made about contemporary ethical practice in the treatment of disability within Western philosophy and popular culture. I go on to outline some of the oppressive and unethical practices which are so often enacted in the 'best interests' of their recipients. The final section of the chapter looks at the impact cultural devaluation has on people with learning difficulties.

Defining personhood

> for practical purposes the word 'humane' means death. It is the polite word linked with gassing stray dogs rather than clubbing or starving them, and with sentencing evildoers to the electric chair rather than burning them at the stake. Wherever that word appears something dies.
>
> (Dunn, in Rose, 1996: 9)

Dunn offers a somewhat cynical appraisal of the real meaning of 'humane'. She suggests that the term can function as a euphemism to disguise acts of violence. There is a well-developed critique of humanism within post-colonial theory which argues that the human subject referred to in liberal theorising does not represent universal human nature but is rather the Western individual subject. The study of non-Western (non-white) people 'expresses a certain will or intention to understand, in some cases to control, manipulate, even to incorporate, what is a manifestly different (or alternative and novel) world' (Said, 1995: 90). The same ethnocentricism can be found in certain individualising approaches to the study of disability. Many of the 'humane' solutions to the 'tragic' lives of disabled people represent a form of colonising of experience. The definitions of person-hood which form the basis of theories of citizenship often exclude disabled people. Disabled people are subject to a different version of the question, cited by Hall, as the most frequently asked of migrants: 'Why are you here?' and 'When are you going back home?' (Hall, 1990: 44). Disabled people are asked 'How did you get like that?' and 'Can you be cured?'. Both questions interpolate an 'outsider', someone whose existence presents a problem to the fully-fledged citizen.

The 'bad old days'

Many Western accounts suggest that in the 'bad old days', disabled people were treated with great harshness and cruelty. Barnes (1994) offers a schematic history of the discrimination of disabled people, the main points of which I shall summarise here. He begins with the ancient Greeks and Romans, who cared for those injured in battle, but practised infanticide on sickly or deformed children. He shows how, in the Middle Ages, disabled people were subjected to a host of superstitious ideas, which led to their persecution. Impairment was believed to be the result of divine judgement and therefore a punishment for sin. Abuse of disabled people was sanctioned by the church. Only 'lately have people with learning difficulties been allowed to receive some sacraments in the Roman Catholic Church' (Barnes, 1994: 12). During the Middle Ages disability was associated with evil and witchcraft. Visits to Bedlam (the first asylum in the UK) were a common form of amusement, and the practice of keeping 'idiots' as objects of entertainment was prevalent among the aristoc-racy (Ryan and Thomas, 1987). During Victorian times, and until as late as the 1950s, social Darwinists argued that allowing the 'feeble-minded' to propagate would bring about the degeneration of the species. Proposals to sterilise 'defectives' were developed and enacted in the USA and Sweden.

Nowadays, the 'civilised world' dissociates itself from such atrocities, and argues that, thanks to medicine, welfare and enlightenment, disabled people are treated with humanity and respect. Like new improved Persil washing powder, we are getting morally better and better. This Whig view of history (Butterfield, 1931: 28) assumes that 'we' are not party to the prejudices of our predecessors.

Sinason has offered invaluable demonstration of the tendency to see the present as an advance on ill-informed and immoral earlier generations. Her research on the changes in terminology used to define people with 'learning difficulties' points out that most terms which sound particularly offensive to the contemporary ear were coined with honourable intentions. The term 'mentally subnormal' originally had no more pejorative intent than the term 'learning disability' has for contemporary users. New inoffensive terms often function as euphemisms, and it doesn't take long for previous offensive connotations to 'catch up' with new 'politically correct' terms. Sinason argues that no one term is intrinsically better than any other. Rather, we need to think about the intent behind the use of the term. The whole question of the extent to which language reflects or constitutes reality is debated in depth in Chapter 7. For now, it is important only to point out that, despite our criticisms of previous statutory and informal categories of disability, these were not consciously used by speakers at the time in order to be pejorative.

Thus, we should not be so confident about the moral superiority of contemporary language. A more valid way of assessing past values is to engage in historical research which assesses the specific meanings attributable to 'impaired people' in previous historical eras. The whole question of the extent to which contemporary society has made an ethical 'advance' in its attitude towards disability needs to be explored through detailed historical analysis, rather than simply asserted. As a number of authors have shown (most notably, Finkelstein, 1980 and Bogdan, 1988), contemporary beliefs, practices and structures shaping the treatment of disabled people may not always represent an improvement on the past. It is worth outlining one such historical analysis which particularly effectively disrupts our 'Whiggish' assumptions.

The freak show

The last freak show in the USA took place at the beginning of the 1990s. However, from 1840 through to 1940,

> the formally organised exhibition for amusement and profit of people with physical, mental, or behavioural anomalies, both alleged and real, was an accepted part of American life. Hundreds of freak shows traversed America in the last quarter of the nineteenth and first quarter of the twentieth centuries.
>
> (Bogdan, 1988: 2)

Bogdan began his research into the freak show with the assumption that displaying unfortunate human 'freaks' for the entertainment of others is cruel, demeaning and exploitative. However, once he began researching the organisation and practices of the freak show, and examining the testaments of performers, he found a less negative picture. In contrast to the assumption that 'exhibits' were people born with unfortunate physical anomalies, who were completely passive in the face of powerful show managers, Bogdan argues that people employed in the show saw themselves as *active* performers who faked or exaggerated their anomalies or differences in order to earn a living. He compares this positively to life prior to the organised display of 'freaks'.

> Prior to their absorption by museums, human curiosities floated precariously, without roots. They existed hand to mouth, lacking the permanence that an organizational base could provide. Moreover, as long as each exhibit remained independent and had only limited contact with other freaks, no community or culture of show people could develop.
>
> (Bogdan, 1988: 30)

Profits on the shows and associated paraphernalia (such as the sale of cards) were high, and were, according to Bogdan, usually split between the show's management and the attraction. Rather than being a triumph of humanity, the ending of the Freak Show marked an end of the celebration of difference and a certain empowering form of 'exhibitionism'.

Bogdan's claims find some support in the story of John Merrick, the 'Elephant Man' who began his working life (after several abortive attempts to earn a living in normal trades) in the harsh and brutal conditions of the workhouse. This was followed by a period of work as a 'novelty' in a freak show, which was succeeded by four years spent in a hospital, under medical care and in sanctuary, where he died. Despite the suggestion made in David Lynch's movie, *The Elephant Man*, that the freak show was a cruel and heartless place, historical records present a different picture (Ford and Howell, 1992). Merrick always spoke well of the showmen, most of whom were supportive and protective of him (Ford and Howell, 1992). For example, 'they tried to devise a padded wickerwork frame to help him lie down and sleep normally' (Ford, 1997: 5). Lynch also portrays Treves, the doctor who eventually offered Merrick refuge in the hospital as a saviour who was sensitive to Merrick's needs and aware of his 'inner beauty'. Yet according to Tom Norman, who gave Merrick his first job as a performer after his escape from the workhouse, Merrick had protested that 'he did not mind being displayed discreetly to a paying audience in the shop, but in the hospital he was stripped naked and felt like an animal in a cattle market' (quoted by Ford, 1997: 6). Merrick only went to live in the hospital following the theft of his life savings, when he was at 'the end of his tether' (Ford, 1997: 8).

There are other portrayals of the freak show, such as in Todd Browning's (1932) movie *Freaks*, which show solidarity and community between the performers and support the view of the freak show as being empowering. Bogdan, Ford and Browning thus offer invaluable correctives to the assumption that freak shows were cruel, and the 'exhibits' were powerless.

However, it is important not to romanticise the freak show, or exaggerate the extent to which performers gave genuine consent or received true valorisation for their performances. Bogdan's account, in particular, is so concerned to empower disabled people by 'establishing their agency and remov[e] them from the category of victims' (Gerber, 1996: 39) that he gives a superficial reading of their accounts, which fails to acknowledge the complexities of their experience. Gerber critically explores the validity of 'consent' and the 'voluntaristic compact' when it is given by people under conditions of subjectification. He identifies preconditions for having real choices, including having a 'significant range' of 'meaningful' alternative options that may be exercised by someone who has relevant 'information' and sufficient 'security'. Gerber shows that these preconditions were not available to many freak show performers because they were denied alternative work opportunities and were 'infantilized, patro-nised, stared at, mocked' (1996: 50). We should not, therefore necessarily take on face value,

> a veneer of co-operation and cheerfulness intended both to make others comfortable around them and to play to some of the posi-tive aspects of the popular stereotype of them. ... One imagines Stratton [one of the performers] and many other human exhibits adopting some of the defensive solidarity and cynical insularity of the carnival world, and ultimately consoling themselves with the thought that they were exacting some revenge on a hostile, insensitive world of ignorant suckers by exploiting their vulgarity and credulity, and rather effort-lessly taking their money. At the same time, we should not be surprised by another state of mind, perhaps coexisting and competing with cynicism. In the narratives of freaks who retro-spectively interpreted their lives in terms of the progress of their careers, we see evidence of the effort to give coherence and meaning to life by seeing it in terms of volition and unfolding purpose rather than oppression and victimisation.
>
> (Gerber, 1996: 50–2)

Gerber suggests a complex mix of motivations, including subjectifi-cation and defensive resistance, activity and compliance, pride and shame, which shape the experience of performing in a freak show. Thus, when freak show performers enjoyed exhibiting themselves, they may have been finding strategies to defend against experiences of pain and shame which became turned around by creative acts of resistance that turned the tables on the oppressors. This point is powerfully expressed by Jim Rose, in the story of his circus side-show of performing 'human marvels' (such as Mr Lifto who hung weights from his pierced body). Rose was born with crossed eyes. He wrote of his childhood, 'My peers would take one glance, start screaming and bolt. Little children pointed to me and clung to their mother's skirts. ... I was a monster. ... They called me names, beat me up' (1996: 37–8). One day, Rose got covered in mud following a storm and found that

> mud is truly the great equaliser. ... You can go up to a huge guy and call him a motherfucker and he's not gonna touch you, because he doesn't want to become a muddy fucker. ... I was no

longer a victim; I was a force to be reckoned with. ... I knew how to amuse peers and transform hostile energy. ... I was a wild kid, revelling in my new hyper, ultra-outgoing personality.

(Rose, 1996: 42)

Although (after several failed attempts) an operation to uncross Rose's eyes eventually worked, he held on to his 'obsession with looking for what gave people jolts' (1996: 47). He'd learnt 'the survival rule of the slickest': to be a 'chameleon' (1996: 49), and to transform himself from the passive and fearful recipient of negative attention to the active and fearless recipient of admiring attention, which positioned the audience, rather than himself, as squirming and uncomfortable. Thus, Rose is making creative use of the defence of projection in order to take an active empowering resistant position against hostile disablism.

Nowadays, the predominant way of seeing those with 'physical anomalies' is through the pathologising medical gaze. A closer examination of the recent history of medicine and its treatment of disability does demonstrate (despite the important caveat made by Gerber) that it is important merely to state that certain opportunities to work and to live independently and prosperously were open to freak show performers in a way that has been denied to many contemporary 'deformed' or 'anomalous' people.

The next section of this chapter identifies some of the ways in which disabled people's lives have been devalued. It identifies a number of crimes enacted in the latter part of the twentieth century, both prior to and after the United Nations international declaration on human rights. Unlike the descriptions above of the freak show, which have identified a complex mix of oppression and empowerment, the value accorded to disabled people in eugenic and utilitarian thinking leaves no space for the celebration of difference. Some of the thinking and practices discussed might reasonably be described as representing a genocidal intent towards disabled people.

Valuing and ending lives

Eugenic thinking

Eugenics is a term coined by Francis Galton in 1883 'to denote the principle of strengthening a biological group on the basis of ostensible hereditary worth' (Lifton, 1986: 24). Galton based his theory on his interpretation of Darwin's theory of natural selection. Darwin wrote in *The Descent of Man* (1871).

> We civilised men ... do our utmost to check the process of elim-ination; we build asylums for the imbecile, the maimed, and the sick; we institute poor-laws and our medical men exert their utmost skill to save the life of everyone to the last moment. ... Thus the weak members of society propagate their kind. No one who has attended to the breeding of domestic animals will doubt that this must be highly injurious to the race of man.
>
> (Darwin, quoted in Gallagher, 1990: 76)

Eugenics is thus based on the desire to prevent the genetic stock of humanity becoming degraded by 'over-reproduction' of the weaker members of the population. There were a range of suggestions for eliminating 'defectives', a category which included the 'feeble-minded', the deaf, the blind and the physically 'defective' (see Rose, 1985). Galton advocated that those who were unfit be identified through the use of statistical measures which would distinguish between standard normal and non-standard categorisation proce-dures. Those falling below a predetermined norm would be seen as being a threat to the future health of the population.

Eugenics has presented itself as a rational and scientifically based theory. However, as many biologists have pointed out, the premise that it is a good idea to prevent certain citizens from procreating, even if accepted, would not necessarily have any effect on the gene pool. Further, even if it were possible to remove certain hereditary impairments from the gene pool, we might find that protective functions against certain illnesses (associated with the impairments) would be lost through selection. Finally, the identifi-cation of an 'impairment' or a socially-valued difference is socially constructed. As Gallagher has pointed out,

> just what constitutes survival, strength or weakness in the human race is a complex issue with many ramifications. The relationship between prosperity in an industrialised society and survival and selection in the natural chain of evolution is not as clear as the first evolution enthusiasts believed it to be.
>
> (Gallagher, 1990: 77)

Eugenic policies have come to be associated with the horrors of forced sterilisation and mass murders in Nazi Germany (Lifton, 1996). However, in their time eugenic theories were supported by a number of progressive social reformers, including Marie Stopes whose work on birth control was motivated by eugenics and Alexander Graham Bell, who was patron to Helen Keller and Helen Keller herself, who warned of the dangers of marriage between 'normal people' and deaf mutes (Gallagher, 1990). The first forced sterilisation of 'feeble-minded' people was carried out in the early years of the twentieth century, in the USA (Kennedy, 1942; Kanner, 1942; Hubbard, 1997). In 1907, Indiana became the first state to authorise the sterilisation of the 'feeble-minded' and the 'hereditarily unfit'. A rising interest in eugenics had led, by 1920, to the enactment of laws in twenty-five states providing for compulsory sterilisation of the criminally insane and other people considered genetically inferior. This continued in some states throughout the Second World War and into the 1950s. By 1958 over 60,000 American citizens had been forcibly sterilised (Hubbard, 1997). Thus, the disablism inherent in eugenic policies was not the product of a minority of racists and extremists, but has become an implicit part of popular Western cultural assumptions. The implicit and pervasive nature of eugenic philosophy in Western society helps to explain some of the extreme violations carried out against disabled people in the twentieth century.

Preventing lives and euthanasia

The concern with preventing impairments through pre-natal screening for conditions such as Down's syndrome and achondroplasia (short stature) has become a growth area within medicine. It is important to consider the assumptions made when an amniocentesis is offered. A positive test often leads to parents being offered the 'choice' of termination. In the UK, abortion is possible at up to 40 weeks into pregnancy for women with impaired foetuses, whilst it is only allowed up to 20 weeks into pregnancy for women with 'healthy' foetuses. Amniocentesis could be used to give parents time to prepare, both emotionally and practically, for the arrival of a baby who does not meet their (socially constituted) expectations. Yet in practice, the assumption that impaired births should be prevented at all costs tends to dominate thinking (see Hubbard, 1997; Asche, 1988). They are sometimes referred to as 'wrongful births'. If abortion is seen as an appropriate response to a foetus with Down's syndrome, then this carries a very strong message to all people with Down's syndrome.

In addition to preventing 'wrongful births', some lives are brought to an end by euthanasia, defined by the *Oxford English Dictionary* as 'a gentle and easy death; bringing about of this, especially in case of incurable and painful disease'. Sometimes the term mercy killing is used. The Nazis based their justification for 'medical killing' on the concept of 'life unworthy of life'. Knowledge of the genocide of Jews in Nazi Germany is well known. The systematic murder of disabled people tends to be discussed less (see Lifton, 1986; Proctor, 1988). Gallagher shows in *By Trust Betrayed* (1990) that the killings of disabled people in Nazi Germany depended to a great extent on the active involvement and collusion of the medical profession. Hitler gave physicians a licence to kill. He writes:

> The people who set up the euthanasia program were not mad-men; nor were they, at least at the start, killers. They were doctors and bureaucrats, efficient men, attempting by central-ised structure, strict policy, and procedure, to alleviate what they perceived to be the burdens imposed upon society by chronic illness and disability. They sought to regularise and rationalise the disorderly state of nature: the life process is so often untidy and inefficient.
>
> (Gallagher, 1990: 56)

> all of the physicians of Germany were participants in the sense that they were aware of the program's existence. They had to be – for all physicians were required to fill out lengthy documents on the condition of each of their chronic patients. Selection was made on the basis of these documents, and patients selected would be transferred to the killing institutions. No doctor could have been unaware of the depletion of the hospital wards or the disappearance of his patients.
>
> (Gallagher, 1990: 62–3)

To what extent were physicians just obeying orders? Physicians who chose not to be involved in the programme were not, according to Gallagher, forced, reprimanded or otherwise harassed. In Nazi Germany we see that the murders of disabled people were not the acts of a minority of crazed killers. The murders were accepted by a large percentage of the population. The killings were implemented with the tacit collaboration of a large percentage of the medical profession (Proctor, 1988). More shockingly, the euthanasia programme continued for over six months after the liberation of concentration camps, and no doctor was ever prosecuted for war crimes against disabled people (Gallagher, 1990).

Eugenic discourse

Hubbard (1997) has demonstrated the tacit acceptance of eugenic thinking in UK and US culture prior to the Second World War. How can the attraction for such thinking be explained? Perhaps one explanation is that contemporary Western culture places such a high value on physical fitness and cognitive function that people who lose large areas of function through an accident or illness or even ageing are often seen as better off dead. TV documentaries debating the human 'tragedies' which lie behind discussions about euthanasia often follow a specific structure:

- They describe the activities and qualities of a person before their accident. Then, a dramatic change is described, which is seen to be experienced as catastrophic both for the person in question and their family and friends. Following this tragic disaster, the quality of the disabled person's life is presented as an unremittingly bleak picture. There is an imbalance between the detailed elaboration of life before the accident and the highly metaphorical reference to life after the accident. Interviews tend to be carried out with non-disabled family members rather than the disabled person in question. The status of relations as trustworthy carers is rarely questioned. This implicit trust in parent, partner or doctor is established by virtue of their closeness to and love for the person in question, despite the fact that children are more likely to be killed by their parents, step-parents or a close family member than by a stranger. There is rarely any exploration of their attitudes to disability.
- Death is presented, following a religious discourse, as a 'release', an 'escape'. Euphemism plays a central role here and the term killing is not used.
- Little or no space is given to exploration of how others have coped with the changes engendered by impairment.
- Often, where deaths are slow, painful and inevitable, the correct use of painkillers can lead to a relatively pain-free death. Hospice care has revolutionised care for the dying. Yet this point is rarely made.

The belief that people should be given assistance to end their lives (and the assumption that some people are better off dead) is often based on the best of conscious intentions. However, such views contain a range of latent assumptions about value and difference which have not received critical reflection.

Quality of life

Utilitarianism

Most people have great difficulty imagining how they would cope if they experienced a dramatic change in their circumstances. It is hard for a non-disabled person to imagine how life would be if they were transformed by a severe impairment. Because impairment is culturally constituted as tragic, for some people, the desire to continue living under such circumstances can seem incomprehensible.

Assumptions about the value of lives often draw upon certain aspects of utilitarian philosophy. The utilitarian assessment of actions in terms of the level of happiness brought to the largest number of people has been interpreted in narrow and individualistic ways which suggest that when people are seen as making a useful contribution to others and achieving a high level of personal happiness, they are seen as valued members of society. When people are seen as being dependent on others, or experiencing high levels of suffering, their lives are often seen as not worth living.

Glover (1990) offers an interesting (and some would also claim chilling) exploration of the problem, in his discussion of the justifications for causing deaths and saving lives. He asks what the moral difference is between killing someone and intentionally refraining from saving their life. In his exploration of the medical justification for abortion, infanticide, euthanasia and the allocation of scarce life-saving resources, he suggests that 'rational' rather than 'intuitive' or 'emotional' criteria should be used in assessing the *total* effects of particular actions and that this should guide decision-making. Thus, we should ask about the costs and benefits to the person concerned, those they are close to and society at large in saving particular lives. For example, in his discussion of infanticide, he argues that where a 'handicap is sufficiently serious, the killing of a baby may benefit the family to an extent that is sufficient to outweigh the unpleasantness of the killing' (1977: 164). Philosophers such as Glover, Singer and Tooley all see the 'right' to life as depending on 'personhood' (Teichman, 1996). A person is someone who is capable of 'autonomous' and 'independent' action. A person with, for example, severe or profound learning difficulties may be considered to lack the qualities defining 'personhood'. As such, they are seen as lacking the qualities required for the ideal and the fit citizen (Teichman, 1996).

Many writers, such as Mailhot (1995) argue that utilitarian thinking, which sees disabled people's lives as being of less value, forms an implicit (although not acknowledged) assumption in medical practice and that, as a consequence, many disabled people live in terror that their illnesses will be treated as an opportunity for 'release' from a painful or difficult life. Research on medical responses to advance directives (regarding the kind of treatment people wish to receive if they became seriously ill or disabled) demonstrates this assumption in favour of ending the lives of disabled and chronically ill people. As Mailhot points out,

> Strikingly, while 7% of the time people got treatment their directives rejected, in 18% of cases they were denied treatment that they had requested. (I got a glimpse of the mentality behind these statistics about a year ago when, hospitalised, I presented my version of an advance directive requesting treatment, a 'Will to Live'. Hospital staff urged me to accept psychological coun- selling because I was not realistically 'accepting death').
>
> (Mailhot, 1995: 14)

Similarly, it is instructive to examine the case of Elizabeth Bouvia in the USA (documented by Pence, 1995), which offers an interesting example of some of the issues involved in assisted suicide. Elizabeth Bouvia had severe cerebral palsy from birth. At about age 30, her marriage ended and she lost a series of financial benefits which would help her gain assistance to give her a certain degree of auto- nomy. As a consequence, she was told that her only option would be to live in an institution. Understandably, Bouvia became depressed following this series of losses, and decided she wanted to die. Because of the nature of her impairments, it would be practically very difficult, if not impossible for her to commit suicide. As a conse- quence, she took her case to court to gain medical assistance in ending her life. The reasons given to support her request were that her severe physical disability made her life not worth living. The liberal press championed her 'right to die' as a human right. Following the publicity of this case, a number of people in the disabled people's movement challenged her claim to be given assistance to end her life. They did not deny her current miseries. However, they identified the cause of her distress in her recent experiences. She was offered support, so that she would not be forced to live in an institution. Following this new opportunity to continue to live independently, and the encouragement given by other disabled people, Bouvia decided that she did not want to die after all. The response of the liberal press this time, was to suggest that she was mad (Mailhot, 1995). This example demonstrates the difficulty which contemporary culture has in seeing value in the lives of people with severe impairments.

Jack Kervorkian (who presented himself as a doctor despite having had his licence to practice revoked) has been a central figure in the 'right to die' controversy. He produced a series of classified advertisements saying 'Show him proper compelling evidence that you should die, and Dr. Jack Kervorkian will help you kill yourself, free of charge' (Marker, 1995: 4). In June of 1990, Janet Adkins, a 54-year-old woman with early Alzheimer's disease, became the first person to die with Kervorkian's help. 'Before arriving in Michigan two days before her scheduled death, Mrs. Adkins had never met or spoken with Kervorkian. All arrangements were made by her husband, Ron' (Marker, 1995: 4). It is interesting to note that the first eight people that Kervorkian 'helped' to die were women, which raises the question of other cultural and social factors entering into the process of 'assisting people' to die.

Kervorkian has suggested that the organs of disabled people should be auctioned after death. Yet despite the ruthlessness which such an auction conjures up, Kervorkian has been described as warm and compassionate. The whole question of whether Kervorkian is a saint or sinner is not, however, the main issue, although clearly many are relieved by his recent conviction for murder. The assisted suicide debate is very complex, and it is difficult to make judgements about the decisions which individuals make, without necessarily knowing their particular circumstances. However, the more general point which can be made is that the debate about whether a life is considered to be 'worth living' should be understood in the context of the social and cultural value accorded to certain people.

The next section examines the whole question of how 'quality of life' is assessed and under what circumstances a life is deemed to be not worth living. First, however, I will examine a more extreme example of the 'death-making' culture surrounding disabled people. There has been much debate (e.g. in the e-mail forum Disability Research) regarding the basis for deciding that certain lives are not worth living. It has been argued that it is not the impairment but social isolation and lack of support which make some lives unbearable. The assumption that certain impairments automatically lead to an unacceptably low quality of life is not rooted in an accurate understanding of the experience of impairment. Rather, it represents a failure of imagination and the pathologisation of disabled people.

The low value accorded to disabled people is demonstrated by the fact that the seriousness of crimes committed against disabled people are often diminished by being referred to as 'abuses'. Specifically, what comes to be identified as an 'abuse' against disabled people would under other circumstances be considered a crime.

> Women with learning disabilities are 'sexually abused' – other women are raped. Men with learning disabilities are 'physically abused' – other men are assaulted. Steal something from someone with learning disabilities and it is 'financial abuse', not theft. … Offenders against the general community are criminals – those who victimise people with learning disabilities are 'abusers'.
>
> (Williams, 1995: 111)

Under such circumstances, Williams (1995) shows that the perpetrators of crimes against disabled people go unpunished and victims of crimes are silenced.

Wolfensberger's critique of the use of the term 'quality of life'

Wolfensberger (1994: 290–1) offers several criticisms of the construct of quality of life (QOL), as it is applied to people with learning difficulties:

- People are judged as having low QOL when they embody characteristics which are markedly different from those culturally valued (such as being judged to be 'ugly', poor or 'stupid' people). Wolfensberger points out that 'under calamitous conditions, such as warfare or natural disaster, almost everybody may cling to life under conditions they might otherwise have judged

to be not worth living, either for themselves or others' (1994: 287), yet we do not advocate mercy killing for survivors of genocide who are living in horrific conditions.
- The term 'quality of life' was developed as a macro-economic index of population welfare (to refer to quality of air, water, social welfare), but it got 'hijacked' for individual and clinical applications, and then deployed to justify medical death-making.
- 'Quality of life' gets equated with 'the value of a life'.

Most people can be quite contented even though they would be said by those who 'talk QOL' these days to have very poor QOL. And vice-versa: people who may rate high on QOL may be very discontented with their lives – perhaps so much as to commit suicide.

(Wolfensberger, 1994: 291)

These criticisms show that the concept of QOL has been used not as an objective value-free measure of the extent to which the needs of a *population* are met, but rather as one laden with cultural prejudices that justify the removal of *individuals* deemed to be a burden. The problems with the concept of QOL open up the wider difficulty of using utilitarian philosophy to justify decisions which 'cause deaths and save lives'.

Criticisms of utilitarianism

The disabled people's movement has been particularly critical of the utilitarian process of decision-making regarding causing deaths because it is based on narrow 'rationalist' criteria which *fail to recognise* the following:

- the affectional bonds between people, and particularly between parents and children, which tend to be unconditional rather than utilitarian in nature
- the trust implicit between the doctor and patient, which is based on the assumption that doctors will not engage in killing. This trust could erode very quickly if utilitarian criteria prevailed
- the difficulty of scientifically calculating levels of happiness. Teichman argues that it is 'impossible to weigh one person's

happiness or pleasure against one's future potential happiness' (1996: 15)

- the problem of how to protect minority rights
- the difficulty of securing 'objective' judgements about a person's worth or social importance.

As Teichman states,

> classifying people as superior or inferior because they are strong or weak (mentally or physically) is arbitrary and unnatural. The man in the wheelchair might be a brilliant astronomer and the class dunce might one day save you from drowning.
>
> (Teichman, 1996: 9)

Often, if someone requires personal assistance in daily living activities such as getting dressed they are automatically considered to have a low quality of life. However, such narrow and technical criteria are of little use in predicting the value a person accords to their own life. A much better predictor for the individual concerned might be emotional well-being or contentment. However, even here, we would never use the presence of depression to argue that certain lives should be ended.

Many of the problems identified with utilitarianism are, in fairness, issues of which utilitarian philosophers are aware. However, it is still important to identify the influence of utilitarian assumptions about the treatment of people with severe impairments and life-threatening illnesses.

In contrast to utilitarianism, Kant argued that morality has very little to do with happiness. Kant argued that a moral action comes from a sense of duty derived from obeying certain universal, rational, 'categorical' imperatives such as 'don't murder' or 'don't lie'. In many ways, the Kantian system of ethics is preferred by some theorists within the disability rights movement because it allows for the possibility of according an absolute value to human life, which should be respected, protected and defended under all circumstances. Teichman (1996) argues that human life is intrinsically valuable and human beings have natural rights. As such, she launches a powerful attack on utilitarian philosophers such as Glover and Singer and their discussions of medical ethics.

Perhaps the central problem with abstract philosophical debate, whether from the utilitarian or Kantian perspective is that general principles regarding the value accorded to people are always shaped by particular cultural, social and relational contexts. The ability to empathise with and value another person often depends on having an ongoing relationship with them. For example, the capacity of a person with profound and multiple disabilities to communicate may only be appreciated by the person or people close to them. This is why attempts to determine quality of life from the outside and then make decisions about the distribution of health and social care on the basis of quality of life are so problematic when placed within an 'objectivist' utilitarian framework.

In the next section, I move on from the question of how a disabling society accords value to particular lives to the question of how disabled people accord value to their own lives. I do this through an exploration of the defences which people with learning difficulties deploy in the face of denigration and social exclusion.

Internalised oppression: people with learning difficulties

Failure to respect affectional bonds

There are a number of ways in which the opportunity to form secure relationships are denied to disabled people. Many of the bonds between disabled people and their families are disrupted by professional intrusions and enforced separations. Mason (1995) argues that even before birth, the relationship between mother and foetus may be interfered with by pre-natal testing, which places a question mark on the continuation of the pregnancy and generates high levels of anxiety. After birth, insensitive disclosure of impairment may create further difficulties for parents in relating to their baby. The desperate struggle of professionals to 'mend' impairments through programmes such as Dolman-Delaccatto therapy, which involves 'forced manipulation of the child's limbs for several hours a day by adults the child may not even know' (Mason, 1995: 2), can lead the disabled person to feel attacked and abandoned by their carers. Generally, the prioritisation of medical intervention demonstrates the centrality of the body as a functioning system rather than the newborn as a relating person with emotional needs which are also crucial for survival and growth. This is not to say that painful medical interventions can always be avoided. However, treatment can become a fetish which inhibits recognition of the disabled person.

When relationships are formed between people with learning difficulties and others, these are often not treated as being important. Research by Hollins (1989) has demonstrated that people with learning difficulties are often 'protected' from the experience of loss by being prevented from attending the funeral when a family member or lover dies or by being denied the opportunity to say goodbye when such a person moves away. Similarly, the experience a person with learning difficulties has when moving into a new institution is rarely explored. The attachment figures of people with learning disabilities, for example carers, are often seen by managers of institutions and services as being relatively interchangeable. 'Basic needs' such as physical care and 'social training' are prioritised above relational needs. Because of this assumption, the opportunity to grieve losses and separations is denied. People with learning difficulties may thus be told to 'cheer up' or be punished if their grief is expressed through 'challenging behaviour'. Such a response carries the message that the pain of loss is unmanageable, since no one is able to recognise it.

Attachment theory suggests that the desire to form relationships is a universal human need (Bowlby, 1973; Robertson and Robertson, 1989; Karen, 1998). When people have learnt from bitter experience that relationships generate too many difficult conflicts or bring about too much pain, they are likely to avoid close relationships in the future. Some of the responses of people with learning difficulties to such failure to recognise their attachment needs are discussed below.

Defences against infanticidal introjects[1]

Analysts and therapists who work with people with learning difficulties have found this client group suffers particularly from low self esteem. In Symington's clinical experience,

> all the mentally handicapped patients who have been referred to me have wanted to discover whether at heart I really want their existence on the planet, or, if honest, would I prefer that they drop off the edge of the world and disappear from my sight for ever.

> (Symington, 1986: 321)

Sinason (1997) identifies numerous cases of her 'learning disabled' clients expressing enormous anxiety about whether their lives are valued. Amniocentesis is a particularly powerful symbol for these anxieties. It is the longest word several of her clients can say and many feel 'that they slipped through because no amniocentesis was booked' (1997: 227). It is often referred to as 'the killing word' in her therapy groups. In the following extract, she indicates that the word is so painful it needed two people to 'carry it'.

> *B:* I agree
> *C:* It is bad
> *D:* The worst word is ... is ...
> *E:* Amnio-
> *D:* centesis'.

(Sinason, 1997: 277)

It is often assumed that people with learning difficulties are oblivious to society's pity, hatred and even death wishes towards them. They are seen to lack the 'emotional intelligence' or sensitivity possessed by 'normal' people. Yet the awareness of and concerns about amniocentesis, which often only emerge after several months in a therapy group, indicate that people with learning difficulties *are* aware of the value accorded to them. However, aspects of this awareness are often not conscious. The pain of rejection is often repressed in order to survive and function under a barrage of rejecting messages. Appropriate feelings of rage regarding the everyday oppression and abuse they endure are often directed inwards, through self-abuse (Oliver, 1995), or in a self-defeating way, outwards in challenging behaviour (Felce and Emerson, 1996).

Secondary handicap

Our intelligence is not fixed and our capacity to think is shaped by the level of anxiety we experience and the uses we make of our mental functioning (Bion, 1967).[2] Freud's notion of an unconscious expression (such as a 'slip') and his concept of 'secondary gain' provide the foundations for Sinason's concept of 'secondary handicap', whereby a person becomes 'stupid' as a way of dealing with conflicts or unbearable anxiety. As Sinason puts it,

> We are all aware of individuals who are highly skilled in their stupidity. To manage always to find the ... worst way of dealing

with written instructions, takes knowledge. Something has to be known well in order to be transformed into accurate error.

(Sinason, 1992: 29)

In other words, a person can *become* 'stupid' for particular (unconscious) reasons, rather than because they are immutably 'stupid'.

Sinason sees secondary handicap as a defence against or, in her more recent thinking, an actual expression[3] of trauma. Secondary handicap involves the defensive 'exaggeration of difficulties' (Sinason 1992: 7). 'The word "stupid" actually means "numbed with grief"'. We are all aware of that meaning in the word "stupefy" ' (1992: 31). She identifies a number of ways in which 'stupidity' can be used defensively to protect the self from trauma.

First, it can be used to defend against the trauma of too much painful knowledge. This knowledge may be of abuse which has been repressed and, as Sobsey (1994), Corbett *et al.* (1996), Brown and Turk (1992) have demonstrated, people with learning difficulties experience higher levels of sexual and physical abuse than the general population. When part of one's intelligence is shut down to avoid certain unbearable thoughts, often whole areas of intellectual functioning are affected. Sometimes, 'stupidity' can function to conceal 'illicit sexual knowledge' (Sinason, 1992: 26). Given the cultural expectation that people with learning difficulties are like 'innocent' children, it can be particularly difficult to recognise sexual knowledge.

Second, people with learning difficulties may exaggerate their 'stupidity'. By making other people think you are less intelligent than you really are, you make them (the so-called normals) the 'stupid' ones. Sinason (1992) describes work with a boy who made himself inaudible. Instead of being a 'victim' of handicap, he handicapped others, because every person who struggled to hear him felt like an idiot. This seems to be an example of projecting feelings of stupidity into others. Another reason for exaggerating learning difficulties is that it makes it possible, in fantasy, to hold on to the omnipotent belief that if you can 'create' stupidity, you can also wish it away. As Sinason puts it, disguising intelligence 'provides a sense of control ...[,] furnishes an omnipotent fantasy that if some of one's handicap can be deliberately created or distorted then the real handicap could similarly be removed at will' (Sinason, 1992). Many of us may exaggerate our shortcomings in order to avoid dealing with the painful gap between our desires and reality. For example, if a person says 'I failed my exam', when they haven't done as well as they would have liked, they can at least hold on to the knowledge that they did better than others realise. Such a strategy means the person doesn't have to come to terms with the painful reality that they have different talents and limitations. As Sinason says, 'it can be easier to behave like the village idiot and make everyone laugh than to expose the unbearable tiny discrepancy between normal and not normal on the human continuum' (1992: 21).

Third, a person with learning difficulties may develop secondary handicaps in order to appease a hostile world. The expression of anger by people with learning difficulties is barely tolerated in contemporary society. 'Racist' myths emerge, to account, for example, for the 'happy' and 'loving' disposition of people with Down's syndrome. Although such myths may be based on real behaviour, Sinason has argued that the stereotypical 'cheeriness' of some people with learning difficulties can be seen as an act of compliance aimed at pacifying a potentially aggressive external world.

> Some handicapped people behave like smiling pets for fear of offending those they are [made] dependent on. ... When people depend for their lives on cruel regimes they need to cut their intelligence and awareness. Black slaves and their descendants in the USA learned to show their intelligence in private and adopt a 'stupid' appeasing way of talking in front of whites.
>
> (Sinason, 1992: 21)

Internalised anger about frustrating, rejecting and painful experiences is thus expressed not just through the way people with learning difficulties violate their bodies, or other people's bodies, but also through their own intelligence (Corbett et al., 1996). One aspect of intelligence involves a willingness to be open to ideas in an external world. The messages from the environment that it would be better if you did not exist can be too much to bear. Sinason writes,

> faced with an internal and external death-wish the handicapped child or adult can cut off his or her intelligence further so as not to see, hear or understand what is going on in a hostile world. Only when we take that on board can we understand better the stupid smiling behaviour.
>
> (Sinason, 1992: 38)

Sinason (1992) has demonstrated that the opportunity to express rage and other negative emotions during psychoanalytic psychotherapy can lead to a marked increase in the vocabulary of her learning disabled clients. Rather than being normalising and regulatory, therapy often helps clients with learning difficulties to become more resistant to oppressive institutional demands, more confident about their own rights and more comfortable with taking on higher levels of responsibility. As such, therapy can help foster a sense of entitlement in those people who have internalised disablist oppression.

Sinason's argument succeeds in linking organic impairment, environmental oppression and psychic experiences. She uses the concept of secondary handicap to explain the complex interaction between these levels. Whilst the term 'secondary' handicap is misleading, since it implies a fixed (primary) biological endowment, which exists prior to experience, it is valuable in drawing attention to the way in which the bodily, emotional and social levels are constantly mutually constitutive. We should not deny the real difficulties faced, for example, by a person with some kind of severe organic brain damage. It is often important to acknowledge, name and respect differences, rather than to try to erase them (for instance, through the euphemisms which are discussed in Chapter 7). Where there is an attempt (for example, on the part of well-meaning professionals) to deny that there is something wrong, the learning disabled client often senses the hypocrisy and is not fooled.

In addition to Sinason's work, there are a number of writers who have shown that trauma and denigration do not only lead to psychologically produced secondary handicaps. There is a growing body of work on the development of the brain in infants which shows that abuse can also lead to physiological handicaps. Travarthen and Aitken (1994) and Fox et al. (1994) have demonstrated that trauma can shape neural functioning. In other words, just as organic constitution can shape a person's experience, a person's experience can shape their organic constitution.

Summary

The fear of having a 'Do Not Resuscitate' notice put on your bed is not a peripheral matter for a minority of dying people. It raises a pervasive fear for many disabled people who become ill, because their death is treated as a 'release' from suffering rather than a crisis which needs to be prevented. If people at their most vulnerable perceive those responsible for their care (such as doctors) to be a threat, the consequences for their sense of security in the world are very great indeed.

This chapter has argued that 'human rights' discourses do not protect all minorities. Since some severely disabled people are seen as lacking the quality of 'personhood' that is so central to Western understandings of humanity, their lives are perceived as less worthy. Medicine presents itself as value-free. Yet in practice it perpetuates a range of practices which betray deep prejudices against those people who are defined as 'incurable' and damaged. Despite the Hippocratic oath, doctors have considerable power to save or refrain from saving lives. Medical decision-making is infused with cultural values. Disabled people (among others, including the destitute, racialised minorities and gay people) have been the victim of what Wolfensberger refers to as 'death-making' (Lifton, 1986), and medicine, by implementing eugenic practices such as forced sterilisation, has played a key role in this. The latter part of this chapter examined some of the emotional consequences of denial of personhood, failure to respect relational needs and murderous feelings towards people with learning difficulties. It identified some of the psychic defences, such as compliance, deployed by people to survive such attacks. Paradoxically, these defences place people with learning difficulties in a position of greater vulnerability to abuse, because they prevent them from challenging their own internalised oppression, and this makes it harder for them to be assertive and resistant to oppression.

Medicine and its allied professions

America seems to be a nation built on the premise that, with great effort and the right technique, there is no mountain that cannot be climbed and no force of nature that cannot go unharnessed. ... Faith in the technological cure encourages belief in the fallacy that all problems have a technical solution.

(Zola, 1988: 370)

One way to close an age is to give it a name that sticks. I propose that we name the mid-twentieth century 'The Age of Disabling Professions', as the age when people had 'problems', experts had 'solutions' and scientists measured imponderables such as 'abilities' and 'needs'.

(Illich, 1977: 11)

Introduction

Medicine's drive to make normal that which it considers to be patho-logical and dysfunctional claims to be value neutral. Yet in practice, medicine contains a series of latent normative assumptions about value, beauty and function which influence its practices. This chapter examines the power of medicine, not only over individual patients but also in operating as a gatekeeper to a wide range of resources and in serving to regulate the health care practices of citizens. It attempts to identify the key features of modern medicine and its attitude to illness and disability. It looks at the influence of medicine outside the clinic, and outlines some of the sociological criticisms of 'medicalisation'. The question of what constitutes impairment and illness is central for medicine since it is only through accurate diagnosis that doctors and allied professionals can identify which

individuals require treatment. The chapter therefore begins by discussing the key features of the medical model of disability that lies
at the heart of most official definitions of disability. It continues by
identifying the way in which medicine silences patients and invali-
dates their experiences. It then goes on to outline the way in which
the medical gaze has functioned to regulate disabled people. Finally,
it reviews those approaches which have challenged the power of
medicine.

What precisely do we mean by the 'medical model'? It is a term
often bandied about and criticised. Further, it is a term which tends
only to be employed by those critical of medical practices. Doctors
tend not to see themselves as 'proponents of the medical model'.
Rather, they see their work as based on scientific understandings of
the body as opposed to heuristic approaches to, or interpretations
of, the body. Given the primacy attributed to medical explanations
and treatment, it is important, before progressing further, to define
exactly what is meant by the term 'medical model'. Bilton *et al.* offer
a useful description:

- Disease is an organic condition: non-organic factors associated with the human mind are considered unimportant or
  even ignored altogether in the search for biological causes
  for pathological symptoms.
- Disease is a temporary organic state which can be eradi-
  cated – cured by medical intervention.
- Disease is something experienced by the sick individual
  who is then the object of treatment.
- Disease is treated after symptoms appear; the application
  of medicine is a reactive healing process.
- Disease is treated in a medical environment – a surgery or a
  hospital – away from the site where the symptoms first
  appeared.

(Bilton *et al.*, 1996: 410)

The medical model draws upon Cartesian principles extended to
regard the physiological body as a 'closed, object-like, physiological
system' (Crossley, 1995), a form of matter subject to the laws of
scientific movement. A central problem for Descartes was how to
reconcile the mind, which has free will and autonomy, and the body,
which is subject to laws of causality. Such reconciliation of the

mind and body is necessary because of the obvious dependence of mental function on the physical substrate.

By seeing the human subject as the foundation and source of all knowledge, Descartes provided the foundation for much Western development – the ethos of autonomous, conscious and rational individuality and the body as a physiological machine. Medicine seeks

> to address the observed lesion, the quantified measurement, more than of a person living in pain. Some theorists, such as Leder argue that Cartesian thinking silences the patient and makes her/his subjective voice become inessential to the medical encounter.

> (Leder, 1990: 146–8)

International classifications

Defining and assessing populations for mental, physical and intellectual normality has become a preoccupation of nation states and international bodies. Perhaps the most widely used and frequently contested international definition of disability is the World Health Organisation's (WHO) tripartite classification: impairment, disability and handicap (Wood, 1981). 'Impairment' refers to any loss or abnormality of psychological, physiological or anatomical structure or function. 'Disability' is any restriction or lack – resulting from an impairment – of ability to perform an activity in the manner or within the range considered normal for a human being. Finally, 'handicap' denotes any disadvantage to an individual resulting from an impairment or disability that limits or prevents the fulfilment of a role that is normal (depending on age, sex, social and cultural factors) for that individual (Wood, 1981).

This classification was devised primarily to recognise the importance of social factors in shaping the experience of disability. Many writers within the fields of medical sociology and epidemiology (see Bury, 1996) regard the WHO classification as a major advance on previous wholly medical approaches. Yet in spite of this (and despite the fact that it is undergoing reconsideration at present), the classification remains heavily reliant on medical assumptions. This is reflected in the fact that the WHO list of impairments is far more extensive and detailed than the list of disabilities, which is in turn more elaborated than the list of handicaps (Ingstad and Whyte, 1995).

It is also evidenced by the fact that the WHO work focuses on the prevention of impairment rather than on removing the discrimination which handicaps people.

'Medical model' is generally used as a term of abuse by Disability Studies theorists. The following section shows some of the problems which sociologists have identified with the theory and practice of modern medicine.

The effects of medicine and dualistic thinking

'Epistemic invalidation'[1]

Given the way in which clinical medicine involves specialisation of tasks, the relationship between doctor and patient becomes a much more distant one. As Bilton *et al.* point out, 'through patient records, X-rays, scans, and now chromosomal profiles, cases can be handled by teams of doctors many of whom may not actually meet the patient in the flesh' (1996: 411). As such, there may be little opportunity for the patient to contribute to the assessment and treatment process. As Wendell (1996) shows, the way people experience their ailments is often not considered rational and is not therefore considered to be an appropriate guide to treatment. Wendell has termed this monopolisation of 'cognitive authority' by medicine as 'epistemic invalidation' of patients' experiences. She writes that medicine 'subjects us to possible private and public invalidation by others ... it has a tendency to ignore, minimise the importance of, or deny outright any of my bodily experiences that it cannot explain' (1996: 122). Wendell points out that scientific research that was initially sceptical of people's accounts often comes, belatedly, to validate them.

> Some people who have a diagnosis find that their experiences of their disease/disability are denied by medicine, because medicine claims to know more about the nature of their physical problems than they do. For example, a small percentage of people with advanced multiple sclerosis experience severe pain in their bones, muscles, and/or skin. Until recent studies confirmed that the disease processes of MS could indeed cause this pain, patients were told that the pain they reported was impossible.
>
> (Wendell, 1996: 125)

It might be possible to challenge Wendell's criticism of medicine. Her recognition that medicine (belatedly) tries to account for the discrepancy between people's accounts and its own knowledge of the body undercuts her argument. However, she is certainly justified in pointing to the prioritisation of scientific 'knowledge' over subjective experience. Wendell shows that medicine has not always failed to accept the validity of patients' accounts.

> When people took to their beds in other centuries, their families, the community, assumed they had a good reason for doing so. They did what was necessary for them. The lives of Theresa of Spain, Florence Nightingale, and Charles Darwin are examples of people chronically ill for many years, but never 'diagnosed'. They were just ill, and that was enough for the rest of the world. But in the twentieth century, if one takes to one's bed and does not seek the medical 'seal of approval' for illness – medical diagnosis and treatment – one is suspect.
>
> (Jeffreys in Wendell, 1996: 13)

Englehardt (1986) showed that (despite being informed by Cartesian dualism), eighteenth-century medicine did not reduce 'pains' merely to symptoms. Pains were considered 'diseases' in their own right, and were classified as such. When 'patient problems came to be understood as bona fide problems only if they had a pathological or pathophysiological truth value' (Wendell, 1996: 183), their 'complaints' came to be treated with a certain amount of scepticism by doctors. Wendell points out that the term 'complaint' itself is instructive in showing how the question of whether their 'real' causes are bracketed. Of the upsetting experience of having your complaint invalidated by doctors saying that 'there is nothing wrong with you', Wendell writes, 'I do not believe that most doctors realise how frightening and confusing such a pronouncement is, how it can shake a patient's self-confidence and undermine her/his relationship to reality' (1996: 123). There are sound clinical reasons for taking the patient's voice seriously and these will be demonstrated in the next section, which will address the following case study of 'epistemic invalidation'.

Withholding pain relief: the case of sickle-cell anaemia

Perhaps the most terrifying form of epistemic invalidation involves doubt about the patient's claim to be in pain. In this section, I identify some of the reasons why people suffering from the gene disorder sickle-cell anaemia fail to gain appropriate medical treatment, and the effect this has on the way they experience the illness. I offer a demonstration of the complex interrelationships between mind, body and psyche. First, it is necessary to outline some of the main medical characteristics of the illness.

Sickle-cell anaemia primarily affects people of African-Caribbean, Mediterranean, Middle-Eastern and Indian descent. It has a one in four chance of being passed on to children when both parents are carriers of the disease. It is called sickle-cell anaemia because the red blood cells become rigid and shaped like a sickle under certain conditions, such as when the sufferer experiences illness, stress, distress, exhaustion, dehydration or cold. Attacks are painful and can lead to complications such as 'strokes, blindness, renal failure, and mobility problems' (Dyson, 1996). The illness is also potentially fatal because of the loss of oxygen supply to various parts of the body (Kraemer, 1994). Yet when not experiencing an attack, the person with sickle-cell anaemia looks perfectly well. Such dramatic changes make sickle-cell anaemia a very unusual illness.

During a sickle-cell disease crisis, the pain is often not taken sufficiently seriously by medical staff. Murray and May (1988) found in their study that a third of sickle-cell patients experienced long delays in treatment and inadequate pain relief. Medical staff often resist patient demands for medication, interpreting such demands as attempts by the patient to 'control' them. Kraemer, in his study of hospital dynamics, quotes a nurse saying 'you can't just give in to him every time he asks for opiates!' (Kraemer, 1994: 203). The effect of limiting the amount of pain relief for sickle-cell sufferers is to leave them in terrible pain.

To what extent is such pain unavoidable? Knowledge developed by the hospice movement, as well as a large study which placed leukaemia patients in control of the administration of morphine, found that when the power struggle over pain relief is removed, the amount of painkiller required is actually reduced (Kraemer, 1994). In other words, the pain patients were subjected to in order to prevent them from becoming 'drug addicts' was unnecessary. Kraemer argues that medical staff should relinquish their control over the administering of drugs, and allow patients to administer their own drugs whenever they choose.

Why, if the evidence suggests that restricting pain relief for people experiencing a sickle-cell crisis is counterproductive, do professionals fail to offer appropriate pain relief to sickle-cell patients? The key reason seems related to the failure of medical professionals to *believe* and then *empathise* with patients experiencing unbearable pain. This lack of belief may be because professionals do not have external evidence of pain that they would have if they could witness a visible injury. Nor can they verify pain. (It is worth noting that until the 1970s many paediatricians insisted that despite their cries babies didn't feel pain, so there was no need to use anaesthetic during operations. The problem of failing to respond to the cries of vulnerable patients has a long and particularly dishonourable history in medicine.) This difficulty in believing patients also seems related to the speed, severity and dramatic nature of the attacks and their abatement. After a crisis the patient may exhibit few signs of the suffering just experienced. Sickle-cell patients' distress is far more extreme than the suffering of patients who have chronic pain. Kraemer found that many hospital staff saw the screaming of sufferers as 'only a performance' designed to manipulate staff.

The suspicion felt towards certain patients is, in part, a consequence of a medical system designed to avoid the anxiety associated with becoming close to patients. Menzies Lyth (1990) identified a number of ways in which contact and communication between the patient and nurse is disrupted in order to keep the patient at a distance, and so avoid the embarrassment associated with intimate contact and the difficulty of becoming 'too involved' with someone who will eventually leave the hospital and who may die. These practices serve to render the patient less 'human' and less of an individual, more a collection of body parts such as (in the words of one nurse quoted by Menzies Lyth) 'the liver in bed 10'. Distancing devices include the development of 'ritual task performances' that dictate standardised responses to situations and leave little room for initiative or spontaneous action. Waking up patients to give them their sleeping pills, ritually taking temperatures and generally treating patients as if they were cogs in a machine may not be the most effective way of delivering care, but it appears to deal with the potential anxiety generated by intimate contact between staff and vulnerable people. Nurses are moved around wards, and follow shift patterns designed to further prevent the risk of becoming 'too close' to patients. As such, sympathy (and its converse, sadism) rather than empathy comes to be the key form of relating. However,

sympathy can only be sustained if patients are able to accept gratefully the assistance they are given.

The sickle-cell patient violates latent rules about 'appropriate sickness behaviour' which require gratitude and deference. The person
having a sickle-cell attack is in such pain that their own needs
completely eclipse norms relating to the sick role. As Freud and
many others have observed, people in pain become totally selfish –
'so long as he suffers, he ceases to love' (1914: 82). As Kraemer puts
it, 'here is an individual thrashing about, screaming abuse at the
casualty staff, demanding a high dose of a dangerous and addictive
drug, to be given at once. This is not what doctors and nurses have
been trained for' (Kraemer, 1994: 211).

Kraemer (1994) argues that when we are faced with people whose
experiences appear to be truly unbearable, we deny the pain. Sinason
accounts for the tendency of professionals to 'shut their eyes and go
stupid not just because it is painful, but because it is unbearable to
see damage and *not be able to repair it* [my emphasis], not be able to
put it right' (1992: 36). A patient's cries make staff feel helpless. The
'difficult' patient, like the disruptive pupil or the assertive disabled
person, refuses to take a deferential stance and therefore withholds
from the professional the satisfaction of being in the omnipotent
position of rescuer. Rather, the professional may well be placed in
the position of the persecutor[2]. Given that many professionals are
drawn to 'caring' work because of deeply personal needs, which are
being met through vicarious care, the frustration of being prevented
from 'helping' can evoke a particularly hostile response.

Whilst the analysis of hospital dynamics goes some way towards
accounting for the failure to give sickle-cell sufferers appropriate
assistance with pain relief, we need to look outside the micro-
environment of the hospital and explore the wider cultural context
to appreciate an important dimension which I have not addressed
so far. This is the role of racism in shaping medical responses.
Professionals often suspect those calling for drug relief of being
'malingerers, drug addicts, and nuisances' (Kraemer, 1994: 201).
There are comparisons here with the treatment of African or Afro-
Caribbean people experiencing mental health problems, who are much
more likely to be forcibly restrained and detained under the Mental
Health Act (Mercer, 1986), and to be given chemical and electro-
convulsive 'therapies' rather than talking treatments (Fernando,
1993). This in turn is paralleled by the experience of black people
within the criminal justice system and in special hospitals. Black

people are constituted as objects of abnormality and suspicion (Parker *et al.*, 1995). Racism has also played a role in the relatively low priority given within medicine to the study of sickle-cell anaemia relative to disorders affecting white people.

Psychological strategies for survival

Patients whose cries for help are not being heard and responded to are likely to defend against their overwhelming feelings of vulnerability and rage by engaging in the defence of splitting (see definition of splitting in Chapter 1). This involves treating the hospital staff as the focus for persecutory experiences, which, according to Kraemer (1994), actually increases the patients' sense of powerlessness. The relatively powerful doctors thus become *all*-powerful and terrifying. The implication of Kraemer's argument here is that whilst racism and lack of empathy provide the main explanation for medical failure to assist sufferers, the patients' defensive response to social, cultural and emotional oppression contributes to spiralling feelings of desperation, panic and helplessness. As their attack worsens patients feel increasingly abandoned. Anxiety makes the pain worse. As one sufferer commented, he felt relief as soon as he could hear the ambulance coming: 'The pain subsides, because he knows help is at hand' (Kraemer, 1994: 205).

Social criticisms of biological reductionism

The implication of the medical model is that all illness and disability, including mental 'illness', is caused by biochemical changes and the fundamental agent shaping human experience is the biological constitution of the body. The logic suggests that if only we could treat all illnesses and impairments, we could eradicate disability. The medical model distinguishes itself from superstition, holism and many psychological accounts of bodily experience because these are not seen as being based on objective scientific principles. The example above of the social, psychological and medical dynamics of a sickle-cell crisis provide a powerful challenge to medicine. In this part of the chapter, I will continue to explore some of the social criticisms of medicine. The best place to start is with Talcott Parsons.

The functionalist sociologist Talcott Parsons (1951) challenged the medical assumption that illness and disability could be fully understood as biochemical malfunctions of an organism. He argued that disability and sickness constituted a specific social role, characterised by licensed deviation from a social norm. The main features of the 'sick role' were:

- withdrawal from social obligations
- exemption from responsibility for their medical condition
- social obligation on the part of the sick person to seek out competent health care as a means of bringing about recovery.

The focus of Parsons' analysis was the relationship of a sick individual to the wider social community.

> Sickness could not be considered merely as an objective condition of the organism without some discussion of the motivation of the individual in relation to the social system. ... Sickness was classified as a form of deviant behaviour which required legitimation and social control.
>
> (Turner, 1995: 38–9)

Parsons was influenced in his concept of the sick role by psychosomatic medicine, which was centrally concerned with motivation in the process of becoming sick and getting better. This assumes that recovery is always possible (Parsons and Fox, 1952).

Criticisms of the 'sick role'

Since the 1960s, functionalism has been challenged for its emphasis on the benefits which social structures have for social integration, harmony and consensus. In the 1960s and 1970s, critics who were writing from Marxist perspectives challenged Parsons for failing to address the dysfunctional effects which some parts of the social system may have for some members of society. The sick role has similarly been widely challenged, for being dysfunctional to some disabled and sick people.

The first problem with the functionalist position is that it relies upon making clear distinctions between the conditions of health and illness, or disability and ability, which cannot be empirically supported. The ailments and impairments that people experience place them along a continuum between ability and disability, and health and illness, which is not clear-cut.

The second problem with Parsons' model is that it assumes that cooperation exists between the doctor and patient, when conflict and disagreement might more closely resemble the actual relationship. The assumption that the doctor should always be trusted is unwarranted. As Frank notes, 'critical and feminist critiques of medicine would label Parsons' worries about 'distrust' as 'the last gasp of a male, professional elite trying to keep its credibility intact' (Frank, 1991: 206). Nor indeed does Parsons address the possibility of medical uncertainty and misdiagnosis (Turner, 1995), although much research has shown that the doctor cannot be seen as completely neutral in their judgement. MacIntyre and Oldham (1977) have shown that a doctor's perception of class, age, gender and ethnicity of patients can have important consequences for the kind of treatment provided, as we saw in the discussion of the treatment offered to sufferers of sickle-cell anaemia. Patients of a high social class are likely to receive greater consultation time. Bilton *et al.* give a graphic example of the influence of social and moral prejudice on medical practice:

> patients ... suspected of being DOA (dead on arrival) are treated in very different ways, according to moral, not medical judgements made about their character – alcoholics, for example, being treated much less sympathetically than those arriving in a sober condition. ... In similar vein, medics in British casualty wards have a private argot for classifying newly arrived patients, including the engagingly named variety of 'T.F. Bundy' (Totally fucked, but unfortunately not dead yet).
>
> (Bilton *et al.*, 1996: 416)

Third, Parsons' analysis of the sick role fails to recognise the role of lay people in defining and treating illness. A majority of patients consult widely with friends, acquaintances and family before deciding to go for professional help. The doctor may be the end process of a complex system of help-seeking among lay people.

Fourth, applying Parsons' model of the sick role to disability is inappropriate, since many disabled people are not ill. This is a point which lies at the heart of the critique levelled by social model theorists at the sociology of health and illness (see Barnes and Mercer, 1996). Thus, whilst social withdrawal might be essential for people with acute illness, extending the notion of the sick role to disabled and chronically ill people may be inappropriate. The sick role is thus not seen by many healthy disabled people as a special privilege that gives them extra latitude to forgo social obligations.

Finally, the rights and privileges which the sick role does offer, are not accorded equally and in the same degree to all sick people. AIDS sufferers, for example, may well be stigmatised and blamed. Parsons was correct in seeing the treatment of disability and sickness as being central to notions of order and normality. However, he failed to recognise that the sick role can have a deleterious effect not only on the disabled person forced to occupy it, but also on the rest of society, which does not benefit from the contribution which the sick person might have offered.

In his defence, it is important not to forget Parsons' significance in bringing the body into his social analysis. Parsons recognised that 'health must be conceived as bridging both organic and "social" spheres' (quoted by Frank, 1991: 206). As such, he provides a useful starting point to an introduction to sociological analyses of disability and ability, health and illness. According to Frank, 'Parsons framed the notion of the sick role within a context of discipline [long before Foucault], but only after Foucault do the implications of Parsons become clear' (1991: 207). In other words, Parsons' analysis of the sick role is not merely a normative analysis of how to deal with those people who cannot fulfil their social obligations; rather, the concept of the sick role offers a useful description of the way in which populations are regulated and made productive.

The medicalisation critique

Following from Parsons' attempt to understand the social rather than the purely bio-medical aspects of illness and disability, the concept of medicalisation has been used to understand the growing influence and authority of medicine. Medicalisation involves the 'incorporation and redefinition of lay approaches towards illness and bodily processes' such that they now fall under the 'medical gaze, defined thereby as a form of illness and open to medical intervention' (Bilton et al., 1996: 430).

Since the eighteenth century, medicine has increasingly taken over the functions once carried out by religion and the law. Doctors have enormous regulatory powers. For example, in the system of criminal justice, psychiatrists may be called upon to assess the degree to which a defendant is responsible for a crime, and doctors are required to validate claims for disability and sickness benefits as well as absence from work. Doctors are an important source of emotional solace and their pronouncements on diet and lifestyle have great moral authority. If one looks at certain life stages or experiences, such as pregnancy or ageing, the influence of medicalisation is most apparent. A range of conditions, which in the past might have been classified within a moral framework and have evoked censure – for example what have come to be seen as 'mental illness' and 'attention deficit disorder' – are nowadays more likely to receive pharmacological treatment. This expansion of medicine has had an enormous impact on disabled people.

In the 1960s and 1970s a number of theorists (notably Illich, 1977) began to argue that medicine functioned as a form of social control rather than as a value-free technology for helping people. They asserted that medicine involves practices that work in the interests of particular professional groups, but that can actually cause damage to individual patients. Five ways in which medicine and its allied professions, in the quest for control and influence, have harmed their patients and decreased the population's capacity to care for itself have been identified as follows:

De-skilling populations

Medicalisation (the extension of the power and influence of medicine to a wide range of activities) has reached such an extent that skills and supports within communities are lost. Medicine intervenes in more and more aspects of our lives. If we look at changes in childbirth practices over the last century, we can see clearly the extent to which this 'normal' life event has become medicalised. In 1937, in the UK, 65 per cent of births took place at home. By 1992, only 1.125 per cent of births took place at home (Hunt and Symonds, 1995). Whilst the hospital is frequently cited as a safer place to give birth, Hunt and Symonds find little empirical support for this. According to Illich (1977), the effect of this increase in medical intervention is that health care has been 'expropriated' from communities.

Treating patients as passive

Medicine has become increasingly hi-tech. Despite the fact that much impairment, illness and death is the result of chronic rather than acute conditions, those areas in medicine which address acute conditions continue to receive disproportionately high levels of funding. This point is particularly relevant to the experience of disabled people, who have received a great deal of funding for technological input, designed to 'cure' their impairments, but much lower levels of funding for the provision of basic assistance. Such practices are reproduced in hierarchies within medicine itself. Those doctors concerned with highly specialised procedures can procure greater status and rewards than those concerned with chronic care needs. There are a number of criticisms which can be levelled at such prioritisation of 'cure'.

Patients are expected gratefully to accept the treatment they are offered and are not seen as having a role in decision-making. Szasz and Hollender went so far as to claim that passivity was a 'necessary condition of good care' (Zola, 1988: 370). It might well be appropriate, during certain stages of a person's life, such as during illness, to become highly dependent on carers. However, for many disabled people with relatively stable impairments, such passivity may be neither necessary nor appropriate. Passive patients are more vulnerable to being objectified; that is, they can be treated 'as a material possession to be maintained, exploited and traded' (Wendell, 1996: 86). Given the specialisation and hierarchy within medicine, patients in hospital can be treated as material to be processed by the system. Hunt and Symonds liken the organisation of hospital birth to the factory production process. They write, 'the shift system, the line-management structure, the emphasis on production targets and the attempts to regularise an unpredictable work-pattern are all familiar components of an industrial setting' (Hunt and Symonds, 1995: 139). Thus, people come to be seen as objects on a production line[3].

Labelling

When a person visits their doctor they may well be given a label such as 'mentally ill'. Thus, according to Goffman, the 'moral career' of a mental patient may be characterised by an initial, contingent 'situational impropriety'. However, 'whether such improprieties come to be labelled as psychiatrically significant depends on such factors as the class background of the offender, the proximity of the hospital and the disposition of friends, relatives and authorities' (Turner, 1995: 74). Once incarcerated in a mental hospital, patients might appear 'mad'. For example, inmates of such institutions may engage in ritualistic and compulsive behaviour. However, when the social context and power relations in the hospital are explored, some aspects of this behaviour can be understood as an effect of institutionalisation (Goffman, 1961).

Inflicting physical damage on patients

the pain, dysfunction, disability, and anguish resulting from technical medical intervention now rival the morbidity due to traffic and industrial accidents and even war-related activities, and make the impact of medicine one of the most rapidly spreading epidemics of our time.

(Illich, 1977: 24)

Illich writes powerfully about the rise in iatrogenic (that is, medically induced) disease and impairment. Some examples of treatments which cause harm to disabled people include the over-zealous efforts of approaches to rehabilitation which adopt a 'no pain, no gain' approach. For example, many survivors of polio who suffered subsequent paralysis are now, according to some commentators, suffering from 'post-polio syndrome' caused by over-zealous 'rehabilitation' work. It is increasingly being recognised that the muscles in polio survivors don't recover in the same way as normal muscles. Intensive exercise designed to build up strength and (so the thinking went) 'independence' actually led to permanent muscle damage.

Psychiatry has similarly been challenged for engaging in a number of 'treatments' which cause more harm than good. One reason for this is that the focus tends to be on *symptom reduction*, which is usually achieved by a general closing down of the individual's cognitive and emotional functioning. The techniques used have varied through the history of psychiatry, from physical restraints, immersion in ice-cold water, surgery and electric shocks to contemporary reliance on psycho-pharmacology. It is worth describing some of the damage caused by these treatments, as delineated by Hill (1983), in a little more detail.

Psychosurgery, used on tens of thousands of patients, involved the removal of the temporal lobes, resulting in a reduction in the patients' cognitive, perceptual and emotional capacities. Electro Convulsive Therapy (ECT) was used on hundreds of thousands of people and entailed applying electric volts to the brain of the patient, inducing a grand mal seizure (epileptic fit) and destroying brain cells with every shock. Between the 1950s and 1980s tranquillisers were the mainstay of psychiatric treatment. Drugs such as Thorazine were used to blockade the neurones that receive dopamine, a substance whose free passage is an integral part of the brain's natural functioning. The brain then tries to compensate for this unnatural intrusion by producing more dopamine. Side effects include drowsiness, impairment of mental abilities, confusion, temporary muscular problems such as uncontrollable spasms, impotence, depression, salivation and drooling, low blood pressure and heart problems. One particularly serious side effect is tardive dyskinesia (irreversible brain damage). Contemporary drugs, such as Prozac, can cause problems of patient withdrawal; Redux and Pondimin can lead to faulty heart valves; Viagra can lead to headaches, blurred vision and heart attacks; Roaccutane can lead to depression and insomnia; and Propecia can lead to impotence.

Despite the above desultory list, it is important to acknowledge that for many people, the advantages of prescribed drugs outweigh the disadvantageous side effects. I certainly do not want to argue that drugs should never be used, since for some people they can be helpful. It may also be the case that a solution to the problem of side effects will gradually emerge with the development of more sophisticated treatments. However, the more fundamental problem with psychiatry is its focus on symptom reduction, and the widespread resistance to other approaches (such as instigating social changes or talking therapies, both of which aim to address underlying *causes* of difficulties). Medicine tends to view the causes of 'mental illnesses' as difficult to change because they are seen as being rooted in a person's genetic constitution. By contrast, a civil rights approach to 'mental illness' would argue that the focus should be on society learning to be more tolerant of people's distress or differences. Systems theory locates the origins of 'mental illness' not in a pathological individual but in a system of relationships (such as family dynamics). Thus, we need to think about the context in which a person is living. Psychoanalysis sees symptoms as being meaningful. We need to give a person space and support in which they might develop insight about conflicts and distress and find a way of resolving it. Removing symptoms prevents the opportunity of exploring causes. Thus, psychiatry may offer some (contingent) solutions, but not necessarily long-term answers[4].

Failing to acknowledge its own aesthetic values

Medicine claims to be value-free and concerned with bodily functioning. Yet the history of medicine reveals an enormous set of treatments which 'improve' appearance. For example, those born with small or absent limbs due to Thalidomide taken during the mother's pregnancy have been encouraged to use prosthetic legs, even when the user has found it easier and less painful to move on their stumps. One speaker at the Sheffield MA programme[5] explained that he had been born with one thumb. This thumb was surgically removed in order to give his hands 'symmetry'. Some Western countries have seen the introduction of 'cosmetic' surgery to remove or prevent the distinctive facial features of people with Down's syndrome (*Changing Faces*, 1998). Disabled people are often subject to a number of risky experimental operations, which can leave them with greater impairments. Operations to 'lengthen limbs' for children with restricted growth are extremely painful, leave patients at risk from infection and are, at the very least, temporarily disabling, by preventing children from activity for many months. These extreme examples show medicine's claim to be concerned with questions of health and function can disguise aesthetic values.

Disciplinary intrusions

Begun's (1996) research shows the extent to which the privacy and rights to confidentiality of disabled people are violated. Grealy's account of one of her numerous medical examinations as a child with cancer conveys something of the alienation of medical practice.

> I was asked to strip down to my underwear, which I did, feeling humiliated and exposed. While the doctor talked to the nurse, my mother and the person on the phone ... he prodded me with his hands, hit me just slightly too hard with his reflex hammer, and spoke far too loudly. ... He got out a tourniquet and wound it tightly around my arm, pinching the skin just like a kid on the playground giving an Indian burn.
>
> (Grealy, 1994: 74–5)

Numerous operations may be undertaken (as in Grealy's case) without regard to the impact they have on the emotional well-being of the patient. Grealy (1994) gives a moving account of thirty operations carried out on her face. All these operations promised a transformative cure that would put right her 'deformed' face. These operations had the effect of putting her life on hold, rather than addressing and helping her adjust to the painful reality of her disfigured face. The 'promise' of aesthetic improvements can have a very high cost, in terms of waiting and suffering. For Grealy it meant that every difficulty associated with feeling 'ugly' as a bullied teenager came to be seen in terms of her face.

Often repeated medical violations can be experienced not just as attacks, but as sexually abusive attacks, making a person vulnerable to further abuse in life. As one disabled adult reported in a survey quoted by Kennedy:

> It did not seem anything out of the ordinary. The way the porter looked inside my nightie and lifted it up and touched me seemed, I think, just like what had been done to me a thousand times before by doctors and other people who wanted to look and prod and poke and talk – all as though I did not exist. All my early hospital experiences 'groomed' me for abuse. If you have never been given the opportunity to object to a doctor taking off your clothes just to look at your leg or if you objected to a doctor pulling down your knickers just to measure your leg but the doctor carried on regardless then how do you recognise that what a porter does to you in a lift is called sexual abuse and that you could/should say no. It all seemed the same to me.
>
> (Kennedy, 1996: 125)

Oliver offers a damning indictment of conductive education, which involves intensive and repetitive physiotherapy to teach disabled people to perform particular tasks, such as dressing themselves 'independently'. These exercises may be monitored and a record will be kept on a particular individual's progress. Yet such militaristic training doesn't allow space for the developing person, who is the recipient of the treatment regime. As Oliver puts it, 'Scant regard is paid to the costs involved in terms of pain, coercion, loss of child-hood, disruption of family life, acceptance of alternative ways of doing things and so on' (Oliver, 1990: 56). Elsewhere Oliver points out:

> If able-bodied children were taken from their local school, sent to a foreign country, forced to undertake physical exercise for

all their waking hours to the neglect of their academic education and social development, we would regard it as unacceptable and the children concerned would rapidly come to the attention of the child protection Mafia. But in the lives of disabled children (and adults too), anything goes as long as you call it therapeutic … conductive education is not regarded as child abuse but as something meriting social applause.

(Oliver, 1996: 107)

Thus, the kind of disciplinary practices enacted upon the physically disabled person (or the person with learning difficulties or the 'mad' person) are much more intensive than those imposed upon the 'normal' (see Goffman, 1961; Laing and Esterson, 1964). The experience, particularly for the infant or young child, of having things constantly *done to them*, often by a series of strangers but with the agreement of a trusted figure such as a parent, can be disruptive to their 'continuity of being'[6], and therefore traumatic. As Mason points out:

Other children play, but you do therapy. Other children develop but you are 'trained'. Almost every activity of daily living can take on the dimension of trying to make you *less like yourself* [my emphasis] and more like the able-bodied. The world is often quite happy to reinforce this.

(Mason, 1992: 27)

Shaming: the objectifying gaze

In addition to being acted upon, the experience of repeated medical interventions involves a critical gaze. This gaze can be experienced as shaming since it implicitly carries the message that the disabled person is not acceptable *as they are*. When the doctor looks at the disabled patient, this patient becomes fixed by the medical definition, rather than an affirming self-definition. Wright (1991) argues that such a gaze freezes spontaneous impulses and causes the recipient of the look to 'become an object' (1991: 31). What does Wright mean by this? It is worth reflecting for a moment on the psychic processes involved in the experience of an objectifying gaze. For this, it is helpful to turn briefly to the work of the psychoanalyst Winnicott on 'mirroring'.

Mirroring refers to the process by which a person is recognised by another. Winnicott explores the way in which a primary carer (such as its mother) mirrors her newborn baby. Winnicott's main thesis is that in order to engage creatively with the world and develop a secure identity, the individual must first of all have internalised the experience of external recognition. As Winnicott puts it, 'when I look I am seen, so I exist' (1971: 114)[7]. If the look of the primary carer lacks empathy, because they have their own agenda (for example, if they are depressed and therefore emotionally unavailable, or if they are hostile), then the infant must put its own needs to one side, lose touch with its own spontaneous impulses and focus on the needs of the (m)other. Such babies are likely to develop what Winnicott calls a 'false self', which needs to protect their 'true self' from a critical external gaze. As a consequence, the person who has not experienced sufficient mirroring may withdraw from an external world that they have learnt, from experience, must be complied with before it is possible to feel safe.

Why is this discussion relevant to the analysis of medicine and its failure to empathise with its patients? Because repetition of an unempathic look, for those disabled children who have been subject to repeated medical examinations, can lead to just such a sense of shame and the loss of, or failure to develop, a sense of entitlement. Medical practice forces an intrusive and powerful Other onto the patient, and disintegrates the subject's 'organisation ... aims and intentions' (Wright, 1991: 30).

Shakespeare (1994) makes the useful comparison between some of the ways in which the bodies of disabled people are fetishised in charity advertising and the way women are objectified in pornography.

> In each case, the gaze focuses on the body, which is passive and available. In each case particular aspects of the body are exaggerated: sexual parts, in pornography, or 'flawed' parts in charity advertising. In each case, the viewer is manipulated into an emotional response: desire in the case of pornography, fear and pity in the case of charity advertising.
>
> (Shakespeare, 1994: 288)

Either way, the pornographic gaze both demeans disabled people and gives non-disabled people a sense of power (Shakespeare, 1994). Similar comparisons may be made between the objectification of colonialised Others. Russo writes that 'freaks shared the same distancing, scrutiny, classification and exchange value as other colonial and domestic booty in the discourses of medicine, criminology, tourism, advertising and entertainment' (1995: 78). For those disabled people who have undergone repeated medical 'treatments', particularly when they involve the attempt to bring about 'cure', it becomes necessary to defend the self against an objectifying gaze. This may be done through withdrawal or exhibitionism. In both cases the humiliation of being exposed is defended against by taking control over how much the Other sees[8].

Many disabled people have experienced repeated violation by medical intrusions. This may also be the case for non-disabled ill people. This does not mean that individual doctors are uncaring, or that certain treatments are not necessary. However, the organisation of medical practice often fails to accord respectful subjectivity to the patient and for this reason treatment can feel dehumanising.

It is interesting to note that Foucault's post-structuralist account of the docile body (which will be discussed in the next section of this chapter) accords well with Wright's existential-psychoanalytic account of 'the look'. The former focuses on the historical context of the fragmenting, classifying 'gaze', whilst the latter described the psychic nature of this experience.

Modifying the critique of medicalisation

Much of the critique of medicalisation was developed by sociologists concerned with examining micro-level interpersonal interactions rather than 'macro' structures such as institutions and policies. The main research methodology used to understand disability was participant observation. Researchers would enter a particular cultural context and attempt to understand the rituals and meanings deployed by people in everyday life. Such an approach enabled the sociologist to empathise with the experience of particular individuals and groups, and also to see the way in which rules governing interactions shaped the levels of control different participants would have over a situation. Whilst the medicalisation critique represents a convincing and powerful challenge to the hegemony of medicine, it is important not to exaggerate the power of medicine. The medicalisation critique should be modified by bearing the following in mind.

First, it presents an over-socialised conception of the subject which positions the recipient of the label as always harmed by medical authority. Atkinson points out that 'the asymmetry of the relationship is exaggerated to the point that the client becomes not the beneficiary but the victim of the consultation' (Atkinson, quoted in Lupton, 1997: 97). Many criticisms of medicalisation fail to acknowledge that medical authority can be helpful as well as harmful. Furthermore, many patients collude or collaborate with medical 'omnipotence', because an authoritative diagnosis (or, to use the more pejorative term, 'labelling') may offer not merely the possibility of effective treatment, but also relief after the worry of inexplicable symptoms (giving external validation of their symptoms). Handing oneself over to an 'expert' may form an important part of the healing process.

Second, the refusal to label people may be used as a justification for withholding services and treatment. This is particularly the case in the field of education, where many local authorities are refusing to identify needs in order to avoid the cost of offering specialised services to pupils with emotional and behavioural or learning difficulties, a phenomenon which is of particular concern in the community care debate.

Third, critiques of medicalisation often over-estimate the passivity of patients and under-estimate the frequency of patient non-compliance and resistance. This can work on an individual level, when patients do not follow 'doctors orders' for example, and on a group level – a number of user groups have been formed to give vulnerable patients mutual support in resisting medical interventions and intrusions (see Parker *et al.*, 1995).

Fourth, medical sociologists have been criticised by social model theorists for failing to address the wider social and environmental contexts within which these interactions take place. Power and inequality are not always visible to the participant-observer researcher, and micro-sociological accounts tend to leave the reader with the impression that the roles of the parties in the medical encounter are the main factors determining outcomes. However, they don't say much about the wider factors which constrain 'actors' in a social encounter. For example, a wealthy and highly educated patient may be offered a different treatment from someone who is poorer and less educated.

Micro-sociological studies have also been criticised for the 'categories' of impaired people they examine. The focus tends to be on those impairments and illnesses which have been romanticised in popular imagery, such as mental illness (Goffman, 1961) and blindness (Scott, 1979). As Bury (1996) points out, more 'mundane' impairments and chronic illnesses associated with ageing, for example, tend to receive much less attention. In addition, until David Goode's (1994) book *A World Without Words* there was very little published work which examined the social construction of severe and profound learning disabilities. As Sontag (1991) has recognised, certain illnesses (such as AIDS, cancer and tuberculosis) have become powerful metaphors for human experience. Sociologists are similarly attracted to the romantic appeal of some severe physical and sensory impairments.

Finally, the critique of medicalisation is increasingly out of date. The high point of medicalisation, in the 1950s, when the medical profession seemed to be above criticism, has been succeeded by a policy change in Western societies towards de-medicalisation. Orthodox medicine is less able to regulate areas of human life as societies move towards community care and de-institutionalisation. The largest growth area in 'late' modern medicine and new systems of health care has been the dramatic expansion in health promotion. The site of medical regulation is no longer restricted to specific institutional settings such as the clinic and the hospital, nor is it restricted to the treatment of a particularly dangerous illness by a narrow group of professionals caring for passive patients. Modern public health is 'preventive; non-institutional; multisectoral; multi-disciplinary; not necessarily requiring the heavy utilisation of resources; and conducted only with the active participation of groups and social networks' (Bunton and Burrows, 1995: 207). In other words, medical and psychological practices are moving into the community. Individuals are increasingly called upon to monitor and prevent disability and illness.

Regulation and the medical gaze

Foucault examines the consequences of the medical gaze for Western society and culture in his book *The Birth of the Clinic* (1976). He documents a new way of looking at patients, which emerged during the move from classificatory to clinical medicine and which he characterises as 'the gaze'. The gaze is a particularly active interrogative form of look, not just at the surface of the body, but, with the increased understanding of anatomy, at the inside of the human body. Thus, the patient under clinical medicine, like the cadaver, is constituted as passive, docile and open to medical examination and intervention. As Armstrong writes, 'the body is an object which could be used, transformed and rendered docile. ... Thus the body was held in, and constituted by, a field of surveillance from which it could not escape' (Armstrong, 1983: 103).

The ward round became a highly significant aspect of medical practice and training, since it enabled doctors to see a large number of 'examples' of specific conditions. The sick person became a spectacle for groups of trainee doctors. Furthermore, the patient was no longer considered as a whole person. Medical care tended to fragment identities through ever-increasing specialisation. Foucault documents the development of a range of new specialist clinics, such as the Moorfield's Eye Hospital, which opened in 1805, and the Royal Ear Hospital, which opened in 1916, as part of this specialisation.

Gradually, medicine required patients to engage in preventive care and (with the development of psychology and psychiatry) self-exploration. Rose (1989) refers to the growth of therapies of self-help as 'governing the soul'. The concept of governmentality incorporates both coercive and non-coercive strategies. As Lupton (1995) puts it:

> Governmentality incorporates both techniques or practices of self-government and the more apparent forms of external government – policing, surveillance and regulatory activities carried out by agencies of the state or other institutions for strategic purposes.
>
> (Lupton, 1995: 9)

Shildrick (1996) demonstrates some of Foucault's observations on surveillance and self-regulation in her analysis of the trend towards self-certification in the administration of benefits. In her analysis of the Disability Living Allowance (DLA) form, she argues that 'the innumerable subdivisions of the questions posed' require the claimant 'freely [to] confess her own bodily inadequacy' in almost fetishistic detail. 'No area of bodily functioning escapes the requirement of total visibility' (1996: 53). Thus, one question on the DLA form asked the claimants how many minutes in the day they require assistance with a number of tasks, including going to the toilet. Shildrick writes:

> The polymorphous forms of domination to which we are subjected are frequently masked so as to appear freely chosen.

Either they may appear expressive of personal desire, or they may be consented to as necessary for individual or social good.

(Shildrick, 1996: 54)

The DLA form thus functions as an expression of power, which involves the continual instigation of self-monitoring. Health promotion plays a key role in the struggle to encourage citizens to regulate themselves. Citizens are presented with an idealised image of human existence, characterised by appearance, 'energy, movement and function' (Wendell, 1996: 86). As Bunton and Burrows point out:

the contemporary citizen is increasingly attributed with responsibilities to ceaselessly maintain and improve her or his own health by using a whole range of measures. To do this she or he is increasingly expected to take note of and act upon the recommendations of a whole range of 'experts' and 'advisers' located in a range of diffuse institutional and cultural sites.

(Bunton and Burrows, 1995: 208)

In this way, the disabled person is made responsible for their condition. This is reflected in a culture which celebrates the 'supercrip' (e.g. the paralysed person who, as a result of enormous will-power regains the capacity to walk). Striving for health is seen in disciplinary society as a moral duty, and patients who fail to take responsibility for following treatment regimens or who engage in 'risky' activities are held responsible for their condition. The effect of this is to blame the 'victim' for his or her difficulty. Health care is pursued with such moral zeal that ill health and disability becomes difficult to integrate within conceptions of community and humanity. Thus, disabled people experience, in sharper relief, the medical disciplinary technologies which are used to regulate all people in modern society.

Summary

This chapter has argued that medicine has played an increasingly important role in the construction and regulation of 'normal' subjects. Specifically, it has argued the following:

• Medicine has made patients passive and visible, by subjecting them to a critical gaze and a range of treatments which can stigmatise and cause physical and emotional damage.

- The normative assumptions of modern medicine remain mystified behind the rhetoric of science and objectivity, but despite this, medicine as a singular authoritative body is perhaps not as dominant as it was in the 1950s and 1960s.
- External regulation seems to be increasingly replaced by the requirement that individuals take responsibility for prevention of illness and disability.
- Interpolating citizens to become *self-governing* has to some extent succeeded the authoritarian forms of external regulation practised in the middle of the twentieth century.

The social construction of disability

Introduction

This chapter introduces some of the key features of the social model of disability which has been the core theory within UK Disability Studies. The social model focuses on citizenship rights and the way in which social organisation oppresses disabled people. Impairment only becomes disabling because of social structures and organisation. Evidence for this is provided by a review of the cultural and historical variabilities that constitute particular impairments as disabling in different settings. In the last part of the chapter, some of the controversies and complicating factors shaping the nature of disability (such as gender and class) are reviewed.

Citizenship rights

There has been a revival within social theory of interest in the concept of citizenship for examining the way rights and responsibilities are conferred on members of a political community. Citizenship confers a set of rights 'both claimed by and bestowed upon all members of a political community ... full citizenship rights are universalistic but restricted to 'insiders' in society' (Pukulski, 1996: 73–4). Alongside these rights, citizens have responsibilities to the political community to which they belong. T.H. Marshall (1950) showed that, despite their apparent universality, full citizenship rights are not equally distributed throughout the population of a state. For example, poor people have fewer opportunities to exercise the social and economic rights and responsibilities accorded to all members of a political community.

However, since Marshall, there have been a number of theorists who have pointed out that his analysis does not address the range of positions and experiences of different social groups (Young, 1989). For example, the opportunities to work may be circumscribed for some social groups, such as women looking after their children. Oliver (1996) has applied a disability rights perspective to the concept of citizenship. Whilst the UK has no written constitution establishing citizenship rights, the protections extended to women and racialised minorities have been much slower in coming to disabled people. The UK Disability Discrimination Act (1996) is much weaker than earlier anti-discrimination statutes. There was initially no commission to secure enforcement and the National Disability Council had an advisory function only. In addition, the Act was full of loopholes and justifications which condone continued discrimination against disa-bled people (Gooding, 1995), such as the broad defence for employers of 'justifiable discrimination', which locates the problem within the disabled individual rather than the barriers in the environment. No such caveat exists in anti-racist or anti-sexist legislation. Whilst some of these discrepancies are changing under the Labour administration (e.g. the introduction of a disability rights commission to investigate discrimination), disability, to a greater extent than 'race' and gender, continues to be located in damaged bodies rather than in discriminatory practices and a discriminatory environment.

Cultural contexts

This chapter argues that disability is neither 'natural' nor essential but rather that it is socially produced. It draws upon social constructionism, which sees the perception of and responses to these differences as being contingent. Social constructionism suggests that 'the ways in which we commonly understand the world, the categories and concepts we use, are historically and culturally specific' (Burr, 1995: 4). For example, the contemporary assumption that to be deaf is to be profoundly disabled is thrown into question when we look at other cultures where being hearing impaired does not have detrimental consequences for an individual's self esteem. The eighteenth-century community in Martha's Vineyard, USA, written about by Groce (1985) illustrates this point.

> For 250 years, deafness was commonplace on Martha's Vineyard. The first deaf resident, a fisherman named Jonathan Lambert, settled there in 1694. He carried a recessive gene for deafness

and, as a result of intermarriage among the i.
this trait spread through generations of Lamber.
... By the middle of the nineteenth century, one i.
of Chilmark was deaf, and in one neighbourhood t.
one in four ... the result was... the entire communi
to use sign language. ... Hearing fishermen would ,
communicate from one distant boat to another. By mid .o00's,
greater mobility slowed the pace of intermarriage, and the
genetic anomaly that created the deaf community disappeared'.

(Shapiro, 1994: 86)

Deaf people in seventeenth-century Chilmark were thus completely integrated into community life, enjoying the same types of occupations, income levels and relationships as hearing people. Social constructionism's cross-cultural and historical sensitivity shows that current assumptions about deafness are not universally applicable. Social constructionism thus shows that our values and ways of seeing are a social accomplishment. As such, we need to focus not on disabled people in the abstract, but rather on the way in which the labels are produced and reproduced in social interactions within institutional and cultural contexts. Knowledge and social action go together. Thus, rather than seeing disability as being a consequence of individual differences, it can be understood as a result of perceptions rooted in social practices which mark out some differences as being abnormal and pathological. Social constructionism has played an important part in problematising essentialist assumptions about the natural body and the able mind. As such, it has been an important theoretical backdrop for critical theories of disability.

The social model and UK disability theory

The social model, as formulated by activists and scholars in the UK, locates disability not in an impaired or malfunctioning body, but in an excluding and oppressive social environment. A number of disabled activists and academics in the UK (Hunt, 1966; Finkelstein, 1980; Oliver, 1990) argue that many restrictions imposed on disabled people are not a natural or inevitable consequence of their impairment, but are a product of a social environment which fails to take account of certain people. Barnes defines disability as 'the loss or limitation of opportunities to take part in the normal life of the community on an equal level with others due to physical and social barriers' (Barnes, 1994). Thus, the absence of ramps can disable wheelchair users. Similarly, 'the inability of the general population to use sign language, the lack of reading material in Braille or hostile public attitudes to people with non-visible disabilities' (Oliver, 1990: pvii) also create disability. The oppression of disabled people has an institutional base rather than being the product of the actions of individual 'prejudiced' people. Instead of examining interactions between people, social model theorists have tended to focus on policy and planning (Barnes, 1994), on the basis that whatever the intentions of individuals, social structures serve to disable certain impaired people.

Impairment is defined by social model theorists (in contrast to disability) as the limitation in a person's physical, mental or sensory functioning. Impairments only become salient and disabling in specific settings.

We tend to take for granted what it is to be healthy or non-disabled. However, our assumptions about normality rely on the articulation of 'abnormal' states. For example, it is very difficult to have a conception of sanity without a concept of madness (see Parker et al., 1995). Similarly, it is very difficult to know what it is to be intelligent, unless we have stupidity as a point of comparison. However, as I will show in Chapter 6, the boundaries between disabled and non-disabled and healthy and ill are not as clear-cut as these concepts might suggest.

Industrialisation and the creation of disability

The whole question of defining normality became a central concern in the nineteenth century, alongside the rise of urbanisation and industrialisation. These developments can be said to have had a role in producing disability and not just because poor working conditions within factories produced many casualties. Mechanised production required a uniform work force, who could perform similar tasks and work was not organised to cater for the range of intellectual and bodily differences between people. This point has been made by Finkelstein (1980), who identifies three phases of historical development which have had specific ramifications for disabled people. In the first phase (feudal society characterised by agricultural production or small-scale industry), most impaired people could contribute in some way to the production process and were therefore included in social life. The proverbial village idiot may not have been respected greatly, but they would certainly have a social role, albeit a somewhat low-status one. In Finkelstein's second phase (industrialisation and the move from small-scale to factory production), disabled people began to be excluded from productive labour. This point is demonstrated by Ryan and Thomas and Topliss, who are quoted by Oliver (1990) in his analysis of the rise of capitalism:

> The speed of factory work, the enforced discipline, the time-keeping and production norms – all these were a highly unfavourable change from the slower, more self-determined and flexible methods of work into which many handicapped people had been integrated.
>
> (Ryan and Thomas, quoted in Oliver, 1990: 27)

> Deafness, while working alone at agricultural tasks that all children learned by observation with little formal schooling, did not limit the capacity for employment too severely. Blindness was less of a hazard in uncongested familiar rural surroundings, and routine tasks involving repetitive tactile skills could be learned and practised by many of the blind without special training. The environment of an industrial society was however different.
>
> (Topliss, quoted in Oliver, 1990: 27)

As a consequence, disabled people were increasingly segregated into institutions and became a separate, special category. In the third phase (characterised by the development of a wide range of new technologies), which Finkelstein sees as just beginning, disabled people will be liberated by the introduction of new technologies.

Finkelstein's account of historical progress sees the major driving force of change as being what Karl Marx referred to as the economic 'means of production'. The means of production includes the social relations of production (who makes profits and whose labour is exploited) and the mode of production (technology). Change does not originate from new ideas. Rather, the motor of change is economic relationships, which transform cultural values and social relationships. Finkelstein's model has many parallels with Scull's (1993) Marxist analysis of the treatment of the 'insane'. Scull argued that the rise of the asylum cannot be understood in terms of humanitarian reforms, but rather that it was a consequence of the social and mic changes which were taking place in Britain at the time. ɪne poor, the criminals and the mad, like those whom we now identify as disabled, all presented a problem to the burgeoning capitalist economy since they were not able to engage in productive labour. They were therefore perceived as a revolutionary threat that needed to be controlled. This control was exercised through institutions such as the asylum and the workhouse, which quickly became a conventional way of dealing with deviants.

Oliver, whilst taking a materialist position, nevertheless modifies Finkelstein's model as over-simplistic in its analysis of the relationship between 'the mode of production and perceptions and experiences of disability' (1990: 29) and as too optimistic about the potential of technological developments to liberate. However, as a way of examining assumptions about the relationship between environments and people, Finkelstein's work is immensely helpful. He clearly demonstrates the importance of economic relations in the production of disability. Given the enormous value placed on work in contemporary society for one's social status, exclusion from work and the reasons for this exclusion provide a crucial key to understanding disability. Despite problems in Finkelstein's schema, it has the value of showing the extent to which our sense of normality and difference does not arise naturally from physical or mental differences between individuals, but rather is an effect of the way in which these differences are framed through an interaction between people in the context of work and society.

The built environment and design aesthetics

The built environment has represented a key area in the analysis of the oppression of disabled people. Several social model theorists are wheelchair users, whose experiences of barriers within the contemporary physical environment played a key role in the development of their ideas.

This section of the chapter is focused less on the way in which environments physically exclude disabled people and more on the degree to which architecture and design are oriented towards the comfort and respect of all those who wish to navigate the built environment. Design aesthetics reflect certain idealised assumptions about the inhabitants and users of the built environment. In different ways, designer 'ablism' is a central feature of classical, modern and post-modern architecture. The stairs, plinths and ornamentation characterising classical architecture serve to exclude the powerless, and demarcate and symbolise zones of privilege. Modern architecture, by contrast, has been characterised as striving towards 'non contextual pure design', based on 'universal laws' of human habitation. However, this approach assumes human bodies conform to a predictable 'able' type (Imrie, 1996). Le Corbusier commented that 'all men (sic) have the same organism the same functions ... the same needs' (quoted in Imrie, 1996: 81). Finally, whilst post-modern architecture does, in theory, attempt to restore human proportions, and reject the totalising impulse of modernism, in practice:

> the era of the so-called post-modern has been characterised by the decline of the public realm, the privatisation of public spaces, the dismantling of welfare states, and the emergence of non-elected local government, all of which seem anathema to forms of political emancipation for people with disabilities.
>
> (Imrie, 1996: 98)

The consequential 'ablist' design has a detrimental impact on all its users, since environments which fail to take account of people with sensory, mobility and learning 'impairments' tend to be environments which everyone finds complex and exhausting to navigate. Steps and badly coordinated navigational aids, such as signs, heavy doors and narrow spaces, often present barriers for older people, those pushing strollers, people carrying a heavy load, people who are feeling tired and those unfamiliar with the environment.

Van Rooyan (1997) shows that inclusion is not just about making buildings physically accessible. They must also be welcoming, comfortable and *readable*. Van Rooyan comments that very complex buildings 'usually attempt to overcome their labyrinthine chaos with hundreds of written signs' (1997: 5). This means that the built environment is difficult to negotiate, even for

> adult, literate, numerate, physically fit specimens, with good hearing and 20:20 vision – the only ones the built environment is really designed and suitable for. ... As an architect, I am often struck how little people register about the spaces they are in and why they feel comfortable or otherwise. In a way, this lack of awareness places the individual in a child-like reliance on the spaces to contain them, as an infant does of its mother

holding environment ... particularly for those who have learning difficulties.

(Van Rooyan, 1997: 5)

Van Rooyan applies Winnicott's (1992b [1952]) concept of the 'facilitating environment' to identify some of the ways in which buildings could be made more accessible, particularly for people with learning difficulties. 'By paying attention to the co-ordination of all the disparate elements, including shape, volume, transparency, incident, texture, colour, lighting, acoustics, and fittings, we can make "readable" buildings which people find comfortable and memorable in use' (Van Rooyan, 1997: 5–6).

Many attempts to overcome the physical, social and emotional barriers to access for disabled people have been only partially successful. One commonly deployed 'solution' is to engineer a series of formulaic adaptations and introduce a system of 'special' access for disabled people. Whilst such 'accommodations' may bring about some improvement in physical access, they are frequently designed, built and implemented in a thoughtless way, which requires the user to engage in a series of complex negotiations to make use of them. Lavatories represent an example of precisely this tendency, and they seem a key signifier of the different levels of respect accorded to people. Admittance to lavatories is conventionally governed by a set of rules regarding one's membership or use rights within a particular setting. For example, in universities, there are often separate toilets for staff and students.

Lavatories which are accessible to disabled people may be locked, vandalised or used for storage. They may be installed in such a way that makes them difficult to use (e.g. the soap dispenser may be placed too high). Often, accessible lavatories lack a mirror and a shelf for make-up, the assumption presumably being that appearances are less relevant for the disabled user. At my own place of work, an accessible toilet was installed with a door which was initially hinged so that it swung inwards. This meant that anyone going past would be able to see the wheelchair user back into the room fully before a series of complex manoeuvres could be undertaken to close the door. This made a particularly private activity public and visible. Such lack of privacy is common in facilities for people with learning difficulties, whose toilets are more often designed for the convenience of care assistants than with the dignity of the user in mind (Van Rooyan, 1997). As Thomas has noted on his arrival for work at a hospital ward for the 'mentally handicapped', 'I was shown the shower-room and toilets – cold floors, high ceilings, glaring lights, a row of lavatories with no doors' (1987: 32). Many lavatories for people with learning difficulties living in residential institutions have gaps above and below the door, bearing closer resemblance to the facilities found in service stations and other public institutions than those found in 'real' homes (Farqueson, 1999). In the past, a single disabled lavatory was often placed in the women's facilities only. Frequently, lavatories which have baby-changing facilities are not accessible to wheelchairs. Thus, disabled people are positioned as people who are not accorded respect, sexual citizenship or parental roles. Adaptations may provide a segregated special form of access which reinforces the position of disabled people as a group who, like the occasional foreign guest, 'we' must remember to think about and lay on extra facilities for. This conveys the message that disabled people are a 'special' category rather than natural community members. 'Disabled' is not a category that cuts across the usage rules conventionally applied.

In addition to 'adaptations' which are poorly implemented and make practical use difficult, accessible facilities often lack an aesthetic sensibility. Napolitano writes about disability in the context of elegant Victorian buildings, that reflect and engender 'a sense of pride in citizenship, a sense of belonging to something larger than self and family' (1996: 34). When adaptations are made to them without any consideration of the extent to which they are in tune with the environment, they reinforce associations of disability as something which cannot be harmoniously included into the 'able' world. Napolitano writes:

> I wasn't at all happy with the idea that getting my share of what goes on in those buildings should inevitably produce an aesthetic blot on the cityscape. If my participation could only be made possible by some ugly contraption, what did that say about me? What would it do to my sense of pride in citizenship? ... Being able to use the environment is about more than being able to 'get about'. At a deeper level it is about a sense of belonging. Until the environment supports mobility impaired people's participation with dignity and pride intact, this sense will continue to evade them.
>
> (Napolitano, 1996: 34–5)

A more fundamental form of inclusion would involve a thorough-going adoption of the principles of what Weisman has termed 'Universal Design'. Universal Design is concerned to produce a 'flexible architecture' based on structures which are 'demountable, reasonable, multifunctional and changeable over time' (Weisman, 1992: 32). This would involve a building design process which took different users into account at the outset of the project. When adapting a building, such a process would be attentive both to the access requirements of a range of potential (rather than just current) users and the aesthetic effects of alterations. Such a change would clearly need to be based on consultation with as wide as possible a range of disabled people. 'Ramps could be constructed in the same stone as nineteenth century buildings and grab rails could be made of brass with elegant Victorian styling' (Napolitano, 1996: 34).

This is not to say that environments can ever be made perfectly accessible to all people. As French (1994) has pointed out, the environment cannot address the access needs of *all* potential users because some people's needs conflict with others. For example, curb cuts may assist wheelchair users but cause problems in navigation for visually impaired people. Similarly, 'some visually impaired people need public buildings, such as supermarkets and health clubs, to be brightly lit, and [some] need the lighting to be dim' (French, 1994; 21).

Despite such difficulty in making environments *perfectly* accessible to all, the main problem is lack of concern about making buildings accessible to only the most 'able'. Examining for whom the environment is built and what messages are conveyed by architectural aesthetics shows the extent to which assumptions about citizenship are built into the environment. The exclusion of disabled people does not need to be expressed actively. It just appears as a natural fact of life. When disabled people are invited into the 'able' environment, the split between ability and disability is left intact. Hegarty *et al.* write, 'there is the tendency to talk of the integration of the handicapped, implying that it is something done to or by the handicapped. Integration is their problem' (1981: 15).

Whilst this section of the chapter has argued that the built environment is central to the inclusion of all people, it is important not to see physical accessibility as a panacea for inclusion. Hockenberry (1996), comparing his experiences in the more 'accessible' West and the less accessible Middle East, found that people in the Middle

East were much more willing to assist him, and this, in many ways, was the most important thing. He writes:

> Once, long after returning from the Middle East, I asked a manager of a Broadway theatre in New York City to help me up a set of stairs to the seat I had paid sixty dollars for at the box office. He looked shocked and told me to leave. If I hadn't brought some attendant to help me up stairs, I could not attend the show. 'We're not allowed to touch you, sir. We're not allowed to do that,' he said angrily. ... This is how things are done in America. In the Middle East, among Arabs and Jews, I would have encountered more steps and fewer lawyers, judges and wheelchair lifts, but I have no doubt that in Jerusalem I would have seen the show.
>
> (Hockenberry, 1996: 263)

Thus, we need to examine not just the material environment, but also attitudes within society regarding inclusion.

The above discussion has attempted to embellish the social model of disability with an exploration of cultural as well as social forms of oppression; for example, the way in which design aesthetics 'stigmatise' those excluded by 'normal' building design.

Criticism of the social model

The social model has been criticised from a number of directions, many of which will be discussed in the ensuing chapters of this book. However, here I will outline some of the key criticisms of the social model which challenge it for its failure to fully address all the complex social factors shaping the production of disability.

First, early expositions of the social model have been challenged for ignoring the differences that various disabled people experience as a consequence of gender, sexuality, 'race', culture or other distinctions. Just as early feminists are criticised for reducing the experience of 'Women' to the experience of white, Western, middle-class women, so social model theorists may be criticised for conceptual- ising disability in terms of the way in which certain kinds of physical barriers are faced by white, Western, male wheelchair users. This point can only be addressed if we look at some of the ways in which disability is experienced from the point of view of people with a range of impairments and social backgrounds. (The whole question of impairment will be addressed more fully in Chapter 6.) Although the social model claims to be a general theory, which focuses on disabling environments, the emphasis is on certain kinds of barriers, particularly those which obstruct people with mobility impairments, at the expense of other kinds of barriers. For example, there is very little work, from a social model perspective, which examines the disabling barriers presented to those who experience emotional distress, communicational difficulties or have learning difficulties. Aspis, for example, has claimed that 'people with learning difficulties face discrimination in the disability movement,' stemming part from the latter group's fear of being labelled 'stupid, thick, mental and mad' by the non-disabled public (quoted in Campbell and Oliver, 1996). Perhaps one reason for this is that the origins of the disabled people's movement in the UK lie in UPIAS – the Union of *Physically* Impaired People Against Segregation. Similar criticisms of the social model have been made by those with sensory impairments (French, 1994). Thus, the claims to develop a 'cross-impairment' analysis of disability actually only represents a limited range of experiences.

Second, the social model has been criticised for adopting many of the values of capitalist society by prioritising work and independence. Walker writes that 'for all the flak over benefit cuts ... the Government's plans for the disabled [relating to new measures to support the return to work of disabled people] ... are remarkably close to what campaigners have been demanding for years' (1998: 17). However, many disabled people who suffer from pain and fatigue see proposals which prioritise return to work (through improving access and challenging discrimination) as also containing the threat of withdrawing benefits from those unable to work. They feel that the legitimacy of their withdrawal from the labour force is put in question (Tregaskis, 1998).

Finally, there have been a number of criticisms of the social model for the way in which it identifies whether a person is disabled or not. In its attempt to avoid medical criteria associated with the nature of impairment, the social model argues that the key criteria for inclusion in the disabled people's movement is that a person must have a positive *identity* as disabled. However, many people with impairments and chronic illnesses would not necessarily identify themselves or be identified as disabled. The only way the social model has of dealing with such people seems to be to accuse them of 'false consciousness'.

The general problem with placing identity at the centre of political affiliation is that it presumes that a person has a core unified self which lies at the 'centre of experience, an initiator of action, a coherent whole, separate from other distinct selves. ... It is presupposed that the self is a unitary entity, a relatively autonomous agent in the world' (Potter and Weatherell, 1987: 101). As I argued in Chapter 1 and discuss further in Chapter 6, self-hood and identity tend, in practice, to be far more contingent and variable than the 'ability/disability' binary suggests. People may have a highly politicised critique of disablism and yet only partially or occasionally identify as disabled. Identifying as disabled may have a valuable strategic function – bringing together a group of people with shared political goals – yet, as Fuss puts it, 'to the extent that identity always contains the spectre of non-identity within it, the subject is always divided and identity is always purchased at the price of the exclusion of the Other, the repression or repudiation of non-identity' (1989: 102–3).

Socio-cultural factors shaping the experience of disability

Disabled people have diverse social and cultural identities, as women, men and children from different social locations who belong to different communities. Disability might be conceptualised as occurring in the 'environment', but its impact on particular subjects cannot be properly understood in the abstract. Rather, it is shaped by people's particular social and cultural identities and their positions. Disabled people share much with those who experience other oppressive forms of discrimination and it may be helpful to identify some of these forms.

Class

Being disabled can be expensive. Access to technical aids and personal assistance can mitigate the effects of and overcome social barriers. Gallagher (1985) in his book, *FDR's Splendid Deception*, showed how President Roosevelt was able to disguise the extent of his paralysis by mobilising enormous resources to manage his image. As Davis writes, 'only an aristocratic WASP could embody the aspirations of the working class; only a physically intact man could represent those who were crippled by the ravages of an economic disaster' (1995: 98).

Financial resources can help disabled people to 'pass' as non-disabled. It is also true that middle-class patients are generally much better served by health care systems than working-class patients. As Jolley and Perry point out

> general practitioners tended to know their middle-class patients better than those of the working class, and to allow them more consultation time. ... [Working class people complained of] failure to respond to requests for information, failure to explain treatment being given, personal derogatory remarks in the patients' presence ... and the ignoring of relatives.
>
> (Jolley and Perry, 1996: 229)

Often, the way in which impairment has been acquired can dramatically shape the amount of compensation and support for rehabilitation services a person will receive. We have already indicated the degree to which social location shapes the chances of becoming impaired. Once impaired, social location shapes the extent to which a person will be disabled.

Racism

Begum (Begum *et al.*, 1994) writes of her experience as the only Asian person in special school and the taunts she received. It is important to attend to the differences between disabled people so that the experience of disabled people from certain dominant ethnic groups (e.g. white English people) is not taken as the experience of all disabled people (Begum, 1992, 1996).

There may be some similarities between disabled people and 'racialised' groups, in the sense that both may suffer from other people's low expectations and prejudices. Just as black boys are more likely to be identified as having moderate learning or behavioural difficulties (Marks, 1993), so people with physical impairments are often treated as if they have a learning difficulty. Further, the intelligence of people with learning difficulties is under-estimated. Racism shapes the experience of disability and the consequences for its subjects are similar. Baynton (1996) has shown how in nineteenth-century USA both deaf people and native Americans were considered by many evolutionary psychologists to be lower down the evolutionary hierarchy because they used sign rather than spoken languages. Baynton notes, 'the power of speech seemed the only difference between reasoning beings and animals devoid of reason' (1996: 49).

The similarities of prejudice against disabled people and racialised minorities are also illustrated in charity adverts where starving children from developing countries or disabled children are most often represented as being more needy, pathetic and dependent than non-disabled white Western children. This point is developed in Chapter 6.

Age

Children have far less control over their lives than adults. This relative powerlessness is further exacerbated for many disabled children, who are subject to extra restrictions that are imposed as a result of various forms of care to which they are subjected. Yet, whilst benefiting the children in many ways, such care can also take away some of their freedoms and rights. Paradoxically, subjecting children to high levels of protection may make them more vulnerable to risks. Kitzinger (1990) shows that panics about children's safety on the streets often lead to new measures to control the unsupervised movement of children. The problem with this is that the street rapidly becomes a no-go area, so increasing the vulnerability of lone children. Furthermore, exerting powerful control over children's freedom of movement may undermine their capacity to develop a realistic understanding of the world. It may also, unwittingly, give the message to those who present a threat to children, that lone children are in some way inviting danger. By focusing on removing the 'victim' rather than the perpetrator of violence, the problem becomes individualised and the source of the problem (e.g. paedophiles or cars driving too fast) is not addressed. Finally, moral panics about children in public places often ignore the dangers in the home, where, statistically, children are more likely to be abused or killed.

Similarly, disabled people have been institutionalised for their own 'protection'. Yet this process takes away the capacity of disabled people to make decisions for themselves, denies them a voice and makes them more vulnerable to institutional abuse.

Many of the issues around childhood oppression and disability are also relevant to older people. As older people require higher levels of assistance, they are increasingly at risk of losing their autonomy and being placed in institutional care. Anthropologists have commented that by neither working nor playing significant roles in the community, older people in contemporary Western societies experience social death before actual death. By contrast, in some African societies which worship ancestors (such as the Nuer), older people experience biological death before social death (Evans-Pritchard, 1940). Miller and Gwynne (1972) similarly argued that physically disabled people living in residential institutions experience social death.

Gender

One's gender is likely to have an important effect on one's experience of disability because idealised discourses on masculinity and femininity mesh with images of disability in different ways. Woman are often constituted as passive, in need of protection, as nurturers and/or sexual objects. Men are often seen as being strong, self-sufficient and predatory. Disabled people are also often seen as being passive and needing protection – particularly if their impairment is associated in cultural iconography with vulnerability, as in the case of blind people (it is interesting that so many 'women in peril' movies involve blind women). They therefore fit neatly with one of the stereotypical womanly characteristics. However, disabled people are often denied the role of nurturer, especially if they themselves are seen to be in need of assistance.

Sexuality

Both male and female disabled people are often seen as being asexual (Shakespeare et al., 1996). This is particularly the case for wheelchair users, who frequently become the focus of prurient interest on the part of non-disabled people. Men in wheelchairs are often constituted as impotent (see Hockenberry's parody of such assumptions, quoted in the Summary, below). These are just a few examples of the differential impact which disability might have on the possibility of a person being seen as a sexual or gendered subject.

Sexual activity and orientation is more closely regulated in people who have less control over their lives. Disabled people, particularly if made dependent on a range of services or if living in residential institutions, tend to have less freedom to engage in sexual activity of their choosing. Carers or parents often make assumptions about the presumed or desired 'innocence' of their learning disabled 'charge'. If a person with learning difficulties is considered 'sexual', that activity is constrained within particular 'normal' limits, such as heterosexual relationships (Corbett, 1994).

What all these forms of discrimination – over class, 'race', age, gender and sexuality – share with the experience of disability is that they place citizens in a hierarchy of power and status. Those lower down the social hierarchy are accorded less autonomy over their lives, are subjected to greater control and are treated with less respect. Disabled people share these experiences with other oppressed groups.

There is much variability and diversity in the experience of particular forms of disabling prejudice. Social model theorists have made a number of attempts, following on from such criticisms, to develop the social model (Oliver, 1996) to account for such diversity. There is nothing, in principle, to prevent the social model from addressing a broader and more inclusive range of disabled people's experiences. However, there are some criticisms, such as the claim that it fails to acknowledge the importance of the body and impairment in understanding disability (Crow, 1996; Pinder, 1994; Hughes and Paterson, 1997), with which social model theorists have dealt less successfully. As Hughes and Paterson point out, just when the rest of social theory is 'rediscovering the body', the social model is reproducing the split between the mind, body and society. They write,

> there is a powerful convergence between biomedicine and the social model of disability with respect to the body. Both treat it as a pre-social, inert, physical object, as discrete, palpable and separate from the self. ... The problem of mind/body dualism is reproduced by the distinction between disability and impairment. The biological and the cultural are pulled apart.
>
> (Hughes and Patterson, 1997: 329)

This critique of the social model accuses it of losing sight of the interrelationship between the three conceptual levels of analysis: the social, psychological and biological. By doing so, the social model makes disability logically indistinguishable from a range of other 'social disabilities', such as poverty or 'race'. If disability has nothing to do with impairment, as Finkelstein (1980) and Oliver (1990) seem to suggest, then there is nothing to distinguish the social model from, say, a Marxist analysis of the underclass.

A core component of the term disability is that it is about perceptions and treatments of bodily, cognitive and emotional differences. What then, is needed is,

> a dialectical approach to the body, which recognises the location of bodies in nature, but also the way in which discourses act to shape bodies, and experiences of bodies, in certain ways over which individuals have only a degree of control. ... Throughout the life span the body is taken up and transformed by social relations, but within certain limits imposed by biology. There is, therefore, a symbiotic relationship between the body and society which defies determinism of either a biological or social constructionist nature.
>
> (Lupton, 1995: 5)

For this reason it is important to move beyond the purely sociological approach, to focus on embodiment, representation and psychic experience.

Summary

This chapter began by arguing that discussion of disability needs to be part of a wider debate about citizenship and social inclusion. It argues that an understanding of disability requires an analysis of different environmental, historical and cultural settings to see how important social factors are in the construction of disability. It identifies some criticisms of the early formulations of the social model for claiming to offer a general model of disability yet, in practice (perhaps unwittingly), focusing on particular environmental barriers that only affected a minority of disabled people. In addition, it argues, certain factors complicating the experience of disability, such as class, 'race', age, gender and sexuality need to be brought into a critical social analysis of disability.

The next chapter engages in further elaboration and critique of the social model, by reviewing critical work on professional power, to show that the notion of 'need' is socially constructed.

Dynamics of care and control

Meeting social and psychic needs

Introduction

This chapter begins by critically examining the concept of 'needs'. It argues that while what come to be defined as human needs appear to be universal and based on fundamental requirements for survival, assessments of needs are intimately bound up with cultural values. Specifically, it explores some of the processes shaping the construction of disabled people as the dependent recipients of care and the construction of non-disabled people as the omnipotent deliverers of care. It then goes on to examine some of the social and psychological interests, pressures and conflicts faced by professionals. Whilst the chapter begins with a far-reaching critique of professional power, it ends by identifying potential points of collaboration between disabled people and professionals.

The discourse of needs

When we talk about someone's 'needs' we tend to assume that these needs can be ascertained objectively. As Slater points out ' "need" is a powerful concept ... because it seems to anchor social claims in the realm of necessity or even nature: statements about need are generally based on assumptions about what human beings or bodies "really are" ' (1998: 316). Professional assessments of the needs of their disabled 'clients' tend therefore to be presented as if they are value-free and based purely on objective evaluation of these clients. The term 'needs' tends to be sharply differentiated from the term 'demand', or 'want', which is treated as if it is based on individual (and possibly idiosyncratic) *subjective* desires, and is thus seen as a 'dispensable luxury' rather than as an essential requirement. It is important to explore the assumptions behind assertions regarding what people need and how these needs are met. Doyal and Gough (1991) argue that the idea of need has been 'widely abused'. They point out that 'on the grounds of their expertise about the satisfaction of human need, planners have justified and implemented disastrous social policies' (1991: 1). This does not mean that there is no such thing as a universal human need; rather, that the concept of human need has been used – particularly in relation to disabled people – in 'authoritarian and paternalistic' ways (Doyal and Gough, 1991).

The discourse of needs thus brings with it powerful connotations, suggesting 'helplessness and passivity of any individual who is "in need"' (Woodhead, 1990: 63). As such, invoking needs creates in itself a strong emotional imperative, which identifies those engaged in critique of 'welfare' and 'charity' as lacking compassion and kindness (Klatt, 1991: 57). The call to meet needs has a powerful ideological pull in contemporary Western society and is often associated with left/liberal welfarist politics. Anyone who questions the discourse of needs is seen as being uncaring.

The social construction of needs

Social model writers, such as Barton and Clough (1995), Barnes (1990) and Oliver (1990), argue that the concept of needs is socially constructed. By this they mean that what comes to be identified as a need depends greatly on social organisation, power and ideology. The disabled people's movement has been particularly critical of charities run by non-disabled people who claim to attend to the needs of disabled people, yet who in practice demean and devalue them. Charity (discussed further in Chapter 8) plays a key role in perpetuating dependency by constructing images of disabled people as helpless.

This is not to say that disabled people are 'independent', but then nor are non-disabled people. All human societies are characterised by *inter*dependence. No person is completely self-reliant since we all (unless we are Robinson Crusoe – and even he had his man Friday) live in communities characterised by the exchange of goods and services. Those people who are identified as being particularly dependent are made this way because social organisation and distribution of resources are arranged in such a way that discriminates against them. For example, if steps rather than ramps are built at the entrance of buildings, then wheelchair users (or parents pushing prams) are made dependent on the assistance of others to carry them into the building. By contrast, if a person 'needs' to catch a train in order to gain access to their place of work, they are not (until there is a strike) considered to be 'dependent' on public transport. Rather, they are seen as being 'users' of public transport.

In contemporary culture, dependence and independence often tend to be thought about in very narrow and mechanistic ways. For example, a person is deemed completely dependent if they are unable to tie up their own shoelace or dress themselves. Rehabilitation training may prioritise exercises which assist such a person to undertake these activities, whatever the cost to them in time and effort. It may well be that a physically disabled person's time is more effectively spent writing than struggling to perform tasks with which an assistant could help. Social model theorists have argued that people's level of independence should relate to their autonomy and control over their own lives, rather than on the ability to perform particular technical activities. Consequently, they argue, their 'needs' are not located simply in their individual bodies. Instead, they are located in a relationship between those whose needs are met automatically – and are therefore seen as having no needs – and those whose needs are not met and who must make a *special* plea for assistance and support. This point has been made in relation to the construction of dependency in heterosexual relationships. As Orbach writes:

> Men's apparent independence ... rests not on their lack of need for others, but on the fact that their dependency needs are in some way legitimised and at least partially addressed by their wives, without their existence being acknowledged.
>
> (Orbach, 1990: 4–5)

We have all experienced absolute dependence during our early life because the human infant is incapable of looking after itself. Perhaps the avoidance of and hostility towards disabled people by non-disabled people is in part an expression of a disavowal of this state of dependency. It is interesting, for example, to note the linguistic association between infantile dependency and illness. Turner (1995) points out that 'the English language does not differentiate between the nursing of babies and the nursing of the sick' (1995: 144). Given this association and the way in which disability within a medicalising culture is treated as sickness, it is hardly surprising that the fear of returning to an infantile state of dependency is associated with disability and illness. In order to acknowledge the interdependent nature of human relationships, many UK disability rights activists have set up centres for 'integrated' or 'interdependent' rather than independent living. This helps to begin to address the fantasies of independence.

Disabled people as responsible providers of care

The work carried out by disabled people often fails to receive mainstream recognition. Walmsley (1994) identifies a number of studies which show that people with learning difficulties often work as informal carers, take on domestic tasks and voluntary work. They often undertake very low-paid jobs which are not easy to fill. This work (like much traditional 'woman's work') is 'invisible, taken for granted, and somehow does not count as work' (Walmsley, 1994: 264). Acknowledging the constructed nature of dependency thus raises the parallel question of the extent to which non-disabled people are reliant upon disabled people. The fact that disabled people are frequently themselves providers of assistance and care, both in their professional and personal lives is often ignored. Morris (1993) has challenged social research – and more specifically many feminist social researchers – for seeing disabled people solely in terms of the 'burden' they present to other (particularly female) carers.

There is growing evidence of discrimination against disabled people being employed in the 'caring' professions. Despite the fact that disabled social workers tend to be appreciated by their clients (Oliver, 1991), discrimination seems to be based on suspicion about the extent to which disabled people, constituted as recipients of care, can also give effective care (Morris, 1993). It is interesting to note that the mistrust of disabled people has infiltrated readings of theoretical concepts as well as professional entry criteria. A good example is found in Bliss's (1994) account of the justification given by her training organisation for refusing her application to become a training therapist.[1] The issues surrounding her rejection are worth discussing extensively, since they raise some of the key 'perversions of practice' that have beset much analytic psychotherapy and psychoanalytic training. Bliss begins by describing the organisation's reasons for rejecting her application:

It was explained to me, kindly but firmly, that severe visible disability in the therapist renders it impossible for the student/patient, who is in a vulnerable situation, to work through the negative countertransference. I was assured that there was no question of my capacity as a therapist.

(Bliss, 1994: 115)

Bliss was confronted with the 'conviction that disability must necessarily elicit pity to such an extent that underlying emotions such as anger and resentment cannot be expressed' (1994: 116). Bliss offers some very interesting case material which demonstrates that the reality of her appearance will always be understood, at the outset, like any aspect of the therapist's appearance or environment (such as their body size, name, dress sense, accent, office layout), in terms of a combination of the particular (unconscious) signification it has for the client and the cultural repertoire which shapes their perception. One of Bliss's clients, for example, felt protective towards her, whilst another looked shocked at her appearance. Both these responses were seen by Bliss as transference responses;[2] they applied feelings from a previous relationship to the current one. The first client had felt that her mother, who suffered from arthritis, always needed protecting. However, after several sessions the client began to see Bliss as a strong and reliable figure, who was *not* the same as her mother. Similarly, Bliss writes, when she discussed his reaction with the client who looked shocked, 'he told me of his secret longing for a perfect world and his belief that all illness and injury were in a way self-inflicted' (Bliss, 1994: 116). Interpretation of these 'transference' responses helps the client to understand what they are projecting not just onto their therapist, but very likely, onto other people they meet in their life. Such analysis of transference is the bread and butter of analytic work. As Bliss puts it,

disability is only one of many factors that may affect transference in any therapeutic relationship. I suggest that such feelings are all grist to the therapeutic mill, as are any feelings the client has about the therapist, and so have the potential to be used constructively, towards growth and healing.

(Bliss, 1994: 118)

The idea that you would admit as training therapists only those people who were constituted as part of the 'mainstream' population and would exclude anyone who might be perceived as 'different' seems anathema to the principles of psychoanalysis. The whole point of analytic therapy is that *anything and everything* that come to the patient's mind should be available for discussion. The point is not to protect patients from 'reality', but to understand the way in which they interpret or project onto this reality. As Bliss says,

> why might it seem so desirable to protect the student therapist so rigorously from the experience of working with a visibly disabled therapist when he or she is training to work with disabilities of so many kinds? If there is an innate fear of disability, of physical difference, might not the opportunity to work with a disabled therapist help the student to confront and work through those fears and preconceptions and thus be an excellent preparation for helping the physically disabled people he or she is likely to meet in practice? And when the disability is there to be seen it can be worked with. When it lies hidden in the therapist's psyche, be it conscious or preconscious, it may prove more difficult for the client to fully perceive and the therapist to fully acknowledge. ... [The] extinction of an anxiety-producing (different) object produces a sense of narcissistic completeness which is in contrast with 'reality orientation and its use of judgement of appropriate action'.
>
> (Bliss, 1994: 117–18)

In other words, Bliss is arguing that her patients' (who are themselves training to be therapists) responses to her visible impairments may provide a valuable opportunity to learn about the way they defend against unconscious fears and fantasies by projecting them onto her, a disabled therapist. Avoiding the discomfort which some people may feel in working with a therapist they consider 'damaged' leaves the patients' fantasies of their own psyche intact. Bliss was told that it is 'extremely rare' for a disabled therapist to act as a training therapist (1994: 118). Given her experience this is hardly surprising.

Whilst the psychoanalytic world has, with some justice, been accused of narrow conservatism, elitism (Frosh, 1997) and techno-cratic immersion (Kovel, 1988), it is probably no more or less vulnerable to prejudice about disability than any other social institution. However, prejudice in the analytic world is particularly dangerous, because the work can be opaque and is generally difficult to assess according to conventional research criteria. Trainees are chosen as much for their personal qualities as academic qualifications and experience. This makes the whole procedure for making decisions about applicants open to abuse. Clearly, what is needed is for all therapy training organisations to have clear equal opportunities policies, and offer training in inclusion and access for all their members.

If psychoanalytic practice, which attempts to adopt an 'open epistemology', is vulnerable to disablist preconceptions, then it is of little surprise that it has been viewed with much suspicion by disabled people. Wolfenstein (1993) argues that psychoanalysis, like Marxism, is an emancipatory praxis, which holds out the potential of emancipatory change. Where psychoanalysis engages in normalising and oppressive practices, these should be viewed as 'the perversion of praxis' (1993: 4). For this reason, it is important to review some of the sociological criticisms of professional claims to neutrality, and some of the ways in which professional practices have claimed to assist disabled people but, in fact, have served to oppress them.

The disabling professions

Professional neutrality?: a question of interest

Until the 1960s, professionals working with disabled people (e.g. physiotherapists, social workers, nurses and psychologists) were commonly regarded as being service providers to the community, governed by ethical codes and committed to the principles of their profession. Functionalist sociologists, such as Parsons (1939), argued that such professionals, in contrast to the self-seeking concerns of the capitalist market, represent institutionalised altruism and community values. However, this unquestioning acceptance of the service ideology is being increasingly challenged. Many studies since the 1960s have discussed the issue of professional self-interest (Lawton, 1982; Hugman, 1991). Disability professionals are no longer seen as neutral. Interprofessional conflicts between, for example, the medical and psychological professions (documented so effectively by Rose, 1985) revolve around territory and power, rather than abstract questions of truth. Illich (1977) has taken professionals to task for misappropriating and monopolising knowledge, disregarding social injustice and mystifying their expertise. In addition to mainstream sociological critique, which addresses general questions about the power of the professions, there has been powerful critique of the caring professionals from disabled academics and activists (Barnes, 1990; Oliver, 1990, 1996; Zola, 1988).

In recent years, a number of user groups have challenged profess-ional authority and demanded changes in practice (Beresford and Campbell, 1994; Barnes, 1996). Paul Hunt's (1981) attack on 'parasitic' professionals and researchers turns the argument about dependency around by suggesting that these groups are parasitic and depend on disabled people for their livelihood. He shows how Tavistock researchers, wearing the guise of neutrality, were motivated more by self-interest than by challenging the oppressive conditions of those they were researching. Davis (1994) develops this challenge by suggesting that the trend towards describing disabled recipients of professional services as 'clients' functions as a euphemism that disguises the maintenance of professional self-interests. The term 'clients' suggests a degree of consumer choice that is not actually accorded to disabled people. It also reinforces the myth that profess-ionals are working for disabled people rather than themselves.

Oliver (1990) has pointed out that the debate between those on the left of the British political spectrum and those on the right fails to address the question of socially structured dependency for disabled people. The left has demanded 'increasing public expendi-ture', which 'will only serve to lock disabled people further into the dependency-creating relationships', whilst the right calls for retrench-ment, which will cast people into 'loneliness in the community' (Oliver, 1990: 96).

Particularly disturbing in this challenge to the 'disability profess-ions' is the evidence that medical students hold more negative stereotypes of disabled people than the general population, and that these stereotypes are stronger when the students are on duty. Diseker et al., quoted by French (1996a), found that empathy towards disabled people actually decreased during medical training and that medical education tends to increase cynicism. Such work is signifi-cant because it enables us to distinguish between the 'goodwill' and 'good intentions' of individual health professionals and the effects of training that focus on treating individuals. These studies seem to suggest that training prepares professionals to treat disabled people as objects rather than as whole people.

Gate-keeping and surveillance

Donzelot (1980) identified the way in which working-class people are subject to high levels of welfare 'policing'. Similarly, disabled people are subject to high levels of surveillance, particularly if they are occupied in responsible or caring roles. A disabled mother who requires assistance with some practical activities associated with caring for her child may find other aspects of her life being curtailed and usurped by a range of professionals. The suspicion of caring professionals towards disabled people is expressed by a woman, quoted by Aldridge and Becker (1994), who commented that 'disabled people hide it [the fact they need help] because they're frightened of losing their kids. I didn't contact any professionals because of that' (1994: 10). Booth and Booth's (1998) study of parents with learning difficulties shows that such parents are likely to be judged in their parenting skills by far more stringent standards than 'able' parents. In fact, their research showed that parents with learning difficulties had their children taken into care for child care practices which were shared by most working-class/blue-collar parents in their neighbourhood.

One important element in the construction of dependency is the control which professionals have over the distribution of services. Professionals play the key role of gate-keepers in the assessment of people for benefit. Medical certificates, for example, are often required in connection with requests for compensation, services or benefits. Parents requiring extra support for their children must obtain an educational psychologist's 'statement of need'. Disabled people are thus placed in a position of vulnerability vis-à-vis professionals. This position has made many in the disabled people's movement sceptical about the possibility of real collaboration based on partnership (Barnes, 1990; Barton, 1989). On the subject of welfare bureaucracies Stone writes that 'keepers of the category will have to elaborate ever more situations in which people are legitimately needy, until the categories become so large as to engulf the whole' (Stone, 1985: 92). Techniques of surveillance are getting evermore sophisticated in what Foucault (1977) has termed the 'disciplinary society'. They require that the recipients of benefits subject themselves to a range of behavioural disciplines.

A classic study by Scott (1979), entitled *The Making of Blind Men*, provides an excellent example of the professional regulation to which disabled people are subjected. Scott argues that the stereotyped

personality traits associated with blind people – such as melan-
cholia, dependency, docility and preoccupation with the spiritual
and aesthetic – do not emerge from any intrinsic difference between
blind and seeing people. He challenges the notion that the blind
'dwell in a world that is apart from and beyond the one ordinary
men inhabit' (1979: 4). Rather, these personality traits are socially
produced. Scott writes that 'The disability of blindness is a learned
social role. The various attitudes and patterns of behaviour that
characterise people who are blind are not inherent in their condition
but, rather, are acquired through ordinary processes of social
learning' (1979: 4).

Homogeneous patterns among the blind population only emerge
because of the way in which blind people are stigmatised and placed
in positions of dependence in relation to the seeing population.
Scott shows how agencies concerned to help 'teach people who have
difficulty seeing how to behave like blind people'. Many clients will
approach agencies for the blind with specific requests for help in
areas such as gaining optical aids and ameliorating practical problems with mobility or housekeeping. The socialisation process
involves discrediting a blind person's view of their problems in
favour of the agency's view.

> Some clients and trainees behave according to workers' expecta-
> tions of them deliberately and consciously in order to extract
> from the system whatever rewards it may have. Others behave
> according to expectations because they have accepted and inter-
> nalised them as genuine qualities of character. The former are the
> 'expedient' blind people, and the latter are the 'true believers'.
>
> (Scott, 1979: 87)

Scott compares such 'expedient' behaviour to 'Uncle Tomism' – a
facade used to appease the expectations of sighted agency workers.
The minority of 'true believers' come to feel dependent and genuinely
grateful. Not all blind people are socialised into the blind system,
particularly if they have sufficient resources and do not depend upon
support. Those who do enter the blind system 'learn the attitudes
and behaviour patterns that professional blindness workers believe
they should have' (1979: 119).

Scott's work looks beyond interpersonal encounters to the social
system that accords benefits to blind people. His work anticipates
some of the insights of social model theorists. Dependency doesn't

exist in a void, but is rather produced by the administration and distribution of social resources, and by the management of relations around the social exclusion of certain impaired people.

What are the consequences of a culture in which specific excluded people are subjected to a range of stringent tests before being able to procure the particular services they need? What are the cultural consequences of perpetual calls for 'need' to be (publicly) demonstrated? One consequence might be to produce what some commentators have referred to as a 'victim' culture. Zola writes:

> in declaring need, people also have to identify themselves as fragile or diseased, in short, stigmatised. The humiliating rituals associated with tort claims (such as postponing rehabilitation and declaring oneself totally disabled) deprive many not only of their rights but also of their just entitlements.
>
> (Zola, 1988: 381)

Interprofessional conflict

A final criticism of professionals is the extent to which their self-interests take the form of interprofessional rivalry over 'patch'. Indeed, this sensitivity can have the effect of making multi-professional decision-making very slow and unhelpful for a disabled person by leading to 'confusion and paralysis for that luckless individual and to a further invasion of the client's privacy' (1990: 28). Disabled people are forced to jump through numerous bureaucratic hoops and to engage in repeated battles yet throughout this process (if they are to avoid being pathologised as difficult) they must maintain a grateful, patient and respectful stance towards professionals (Marks, 1996b).

So far, the criticisms outlined above have not differentiated between different professional groups and can thus be accused of unjustifiably tarring all professionals with the same brush. In fact, professional cultures vary enormously in the extent to which they accord respect, autonomy and power to disabled people. The emphasis placed by social model theorists on professional self-interest might be experienced as particularly galling for those nurses who work in the British National Health Service, many of whom feel that their low wages are a form of exploitation and that they have little control over the organisation of their work. Similarly, emancipatory practices are fostered by some educational psychologists, who engage in battles with schools to secure inclusion for pupils the schools insist cannot be managed within a mainstream context. Some schools are striving to make themselves fully inclusive, whilst some social workers are involved in and supportive of disability equality training and the full implementation of equal opportunities policies. In other words, some of the conflicts between professionals identified above actually position some professionals as allies of disabled people.

Perhaps the failure to acknowledge differences between professionals in social model accounts reflects the desire to see disabled people from different impairment, social and age groups as one unified group[3]. However, lumping professionals together as the uniform 'enemy' may, as the next section of this chapter argues, be counter-productive in forming alliances to challenge disabling barriers. One reason for this is that the discourse of the disabling professions can be alienating and can give professionals the message that whatever they do, they are going to be objects of suspicion. For this reason the next section attempts to look not only at the oppressive practices in which many professionals engage, but also at some of the constraints placed on specific professional groups, which result in disablism.

'Disabled' professionals

This section identifies some of the political and psychological pressures which shape professional practice. Having recognised the need for a certain amount of scepticism towards professional claims regarding their 'disinterested' service orientation, it is important not to go too far the other way, and reduce all professional activities to narrow self-interest. Simplistic demonisation of professionals fails to recognise the external constraints placed on them or to distinguish between 'good intentions' and damaging cultures and practices. This part of the chapter therefore attempts not to condemn but to account for the roots of disablism.

Professionals mirror clients

In many ways, the position of self-regulating professionals mirrors the position of their clients. The erosion of automatic trust in professionals may seem justified given the criticisms made earlier in this chapter. However, attempting to remedy this by regulation (i.e. a culture of increasingly bureaucratic monitoring of professionals) can be damaging to morale without necessarily improving the situation of the recipients of services. We are living in a culture that demands constant change and 'improvement'. Perpetual re-evaluation of professional practice has led to what Obholzer and Roberts (1994) describe as 'manic reorganisation' of services, both in the British National Health Service and in the voluntary sector. Financial restrictions increase the pressures placed on professionals by generating ever-higher levels of work. Oliver (1991) rightly points out that professionals face numerous barriers to bringing about effective change.

Further, the value accorded to professionals and carers/assistants seems to mirror the value accorded to the people they work with. This can be expressed in several ways. Those working most closely with disabled people experience related forms of stigma. As Goffman puts it, the 'loyal spouse of the mental patient, the daughter of the ex-con, the parent of the cripple [sic] ... share some of the discredit of the stigmatised person' (1963: 43). Those working in the field of disability tend to be offered fewer opportunities for advancement and poorer working conditions.

This point is demonstrated by research carried out by Marks *et al.* (1998) on the 'training needs' of staff working in a low-secure unit for people with learning difficulties and challenging behaviour. The study showed that staff experienced much of the isolation and denigration felt by clients. A particular area of staff dissatisfaction concerned the lack of training in work with such a vulnerable and difficult[4] client group. One support worker expressed an interest in taking a National Vocational Qualification. He had been promised this opportunity by the managers of the service, but it had never materialised. This member of staff commented, 'there's not a lot of praise. It's just, like, get on with it. ... We've not had any teaching sessions or anything. And when it comes to having them they are not followed through' (Marks *et al.*, 1998: 30). Many of the support workers in the unit felt that they were treated (like the learning disabled clients) as if they were 'stupid'. One of the few areas in which they did feel valued was through the exercise of physical control in the 'control and restraint' training they had received. It is therefore not surprising that they had far less confidence in their ability to form relationships with clients than in their ability to control them, sometimes to the point of committing acts of physical abuse.

The value accorded to professionals and support workers who

have closest contact with disabled people is also reflected in the levels of remuneration offered. Even within the prestigious profession of medicine, those doctors working in the area of mental health, learning disability and gerontology (all of which are concerned to a great extent with disabling impairments) tend to be accorded lower status than doctors working within more 'glamorous' specialist areas such as surgery, which are not associated with a particular devalued social group (Marks *et al.*, 1998).

The mirroring relationships between 'disability' professionals and 'clients' is expressed particularly clearly in a paper by Lawton (1982) on the history of social work. He sees professional altruism as a myth. In Skynner's (1991) summary of Lawton's paper a particularly bleak picture is presented of the social work profession in which

> [many] public service agencies dealing with the most deprived and disadvantaged clients are themselves demoralised and unsupported. They resist change, show high turnover in the senior administration, are unsupportive to their case-workers, are secretive and restrict communication, are controlling in an infantilising way, are rigidly bureaucratic, value conformity but dislike opposition or criticism; they 'use' their social workers rather than respect them as persons, demand loyalty to their organisation at the expense of encouraging the search for adequate training, and they generate rage in the workers but force them to suppress it ... case workers can be comforted by the realisation that their clients are even more miserably served than themselves and do in fact derive little comfort, even from them.
>
> (Skynner, 1991: 160)

In other words, professionals working closely with disabled people and other oppressed groups may 'pass' the devaluation and stress of their work onto their clients. Yet at the same time as identifying with clients' difficulties, the anxiety of coming into contact with people experiencing difficulties or suffering can be dealt with by employing a range of what Menzies Lyth (1990) calls 'institutional defence mechanisms' (which were discussed in Chapter 3). For example, one way of dealing with the stresses of working in the medium-secure unit for 'challenging' clients was to engage in 'emotional distancing'. As one support worker said, 'you do try and cut yourself off but it's very difficult' (quoted in Marks *et al.*, 1998: 40). However, this strategy led many staff to feel guilt about not giving 'one hundred per cent' (1998: 42). Similar processes have been identified in studies of psychiatric nurses. As Bott Spillius writes,

> Since nurses cannot get away from the madness physically, they get away from it emotionally; they develop some form of relationship that locates madness in the patient and sanity in themselves, with a barrier to prevent contamination. ... Such an arrangement allows the nurses to stay in the situation without feeling that their minds are being damaged. ... Talking to patients is dangerous because it threatens to puncture the barrier that keeps sanity and madness in their proper places.
>
> (Bott Spillius, 1990: 604–5)

Without structured supervision giving staff a space in which to process their experiences of working with an oppressed and often understandably depressed client group, emotional withdrawal may be the only strategy available for surviving at work.

Vicarious care

In addition to dealing with organisational frustrations, anxieties and cultural devaluation, those people who choose to work with a client group that is highly stigmatised are likely to have low self esteem, like their clients (Shapiro and Carr, 1991). This may be because people are often drawn to working with those groups of people with whom they in some way (possibly unconsciously) identify. As Skynner puts it:

> The mental health professional automatically selects the ideal clientele in which to study himself or herself vicariously and discover what is missing ... though the knowledge cannot benefit us ... until we acknowledge the fact that our work, however useful, has also been an evasion of the truth about ourselves. ... I'll look after you if you'll look after the bit of me I can't look after.
>
> (Skynner, 1991: xviii)

In other words, the person who is unable to deal with their own rage, vulnerability or sense of shame may identify these characteristics in others, and remain connected with these disowned parts of themselves, through contact with stigmatised people. The institutional stresses and personal investments which many professionals experience thus often serve to disempower their clients. This section of the chapter has argued that it is important to recognise that the whole process of providing 'care' is a complex social accomplishment, involving a range of cultural and psychological factors. The social value accorded to disabled people is mirrored by the social value accorded to people providing 'services' for them. Furthermore, lack of social recognition and respect reinforces low self esteem, internalised oppression and the desire to locate one's own psychological difficulties elsewhere.

Fostering collaboration between professionals and disabled people

A rehabilitation/independent living compact

Having identified a series of difficulties which the 'disabled'/'disabling' professions have in their relations with each other, with themselves and subsequently with clients, this part of the chapter explores some ways of fostering shared interests and forming new alliances. De Jong (1993) argues that it is in the interests of professionals to become allies to the disabled people's movement. Currently, many professionals see disabled people's demands for civil rights and autonomy in decision-making as a threat to their authority. However by holding themselves up as sole experts, professionals lay themselves open to scapegoating when they are unable to deliver effective help for their clients. De Jong states that it is in the long-term interests of the rehabilitation profession to ally itself to the independent living movement, and obtain goodwill and contacts in the community. Both the independent living movement and rehabilitation professionals will benefit from collaboration. De Jong points out, 'rehabilitation facilities need to look to the expertise that the consumer community can give to improve a facility's own programs and services' (1993: 1022). Similarly, the independent living/disability rights movement could benefit from the enormous resources in financial and personnel management and marketing skills 'that can help a new Independent Living Centre get off the ground' (1993: 1022.). De Jong argues that a new compact is needed, one that is based on the notion of social obligation and democratic collaboration between professionals and activists, and that will benefit both groups.

Psychologists and therapists as allies and advocates

There are a number of examples of organisations of professionals and disabled people working collaboratively. One of the most radical of these groups is Psychology, Politics and Resistance, which is a network of psychologists and non-psychologists (including survivors of the mental health system) who 'are committed to challenging the oppressive use of psychological ideas, supporting those on the receiving end, and using psychological knowledge positively to help those engaged in struggles for social justice' (*PPR Newsletter*, 1998). Others offer services which are empowering and sensitive to service users. For example, the Afro-Caribbean Mental Health Project, based in Brixton, encourages mental health services to becomes more sensitive to the needs of the African-Caribbean community[5] .Finally, there are many groups of people (such as Parents as Partner and Disability Equality in Education) which have close relationships with disabled people (and include 'carers'). They identify themselves primarily as allies working alongside (rather than for) disabled people in order to challenge disabling barriers.

Returning to some of the analytic psychotherapists we have discussed in this book, there are also some important examples of psychotherapists moving out of the consulting room to act as allies to disabled people. Kraemer, the psychoanalytic psychotherapist who carried out a study of the treatment of sickle-cell patients (discussed in Chapter 3), become an advocate for sickle-cell sufferers and a campaigner to bring about change in professional practices, rather than merely describing the health system, or assisting the boy he was working with to understand his 'persecutory fears'. He was concerned first and foremost not to help patients feel 'calmer' and adjust to the horrors of their attacks, but rather to empower patients by challenging the racist system which withholds sufficient pain relief medication. As such, Kraemer's work represents an important politicised style of action research, which succeeds in integrating a critical analysis of local professional practices and wider social structures with an appreciation of the physiological and psychic experiences not just of patients but of the health care system. Similarly, Sinason (1992) working in the field of learning disability is a long-standing ally in campaigns to gain sexual rights for people with learning difficulties. Such recognition of the need to address both the internal and external world of their clients seems important to avoid, on the one hand, pathologising individuals and, on the other, failing to recognise their emotional experiences.

I am not suggesting that all therapists give up their day job, and become advocates or allies. However, I am arguing that those people engaged in attempting to understand the inner world of the people they work with would improve their work if they became politically literate regarding the social experiences of the broad range of social groups with which they come into contact.

Summary

This chapter argues that it is important to assess critically *both* the material and the psychological investments of those who work to 'help' disabled people. It challenges the 'service' ideology that portrays professionals as disinterested, following social model theorists who have shown that 'needs' and 'care' are socially constructed. Yet it also argues that some of the oppressive ways in which professionals behave are a product of the cultural and institutional pressures which they face. If professionals were able to acknowledge and own their investments in disability more openly and, it might become possible to engage in real collaboration that benefits everyone. As Schlapobersky puts it, 'if professionals can include themselves in the equation of change, a process of mutual growth and learning ensues, bringing personal benefits to both sides' (Schlapobersky, 1991: xiv). In this way, disabled people and those who work with them are *not* engaged in

> a zero sum equation where the less I gain the more there is for others. [Rather] [t]he more I gain, the more there is for them, and vice versa. ... The more each of us gains the more there is for everyone.
>
> (Skynner, 1991: xiv)

Whilst this scenario of mutual gain may sound a trifle over-optimistic and it remains important for disabled people to challenge professional arrogance and oppressive practices, it is also important not to reduce the relationship between disabled people and professionals to one characterised simply by conflict and 'parasitism' (see Hunt, 1981). Rather, as De Jong and Skynner have argued, it is important to explore the possibilities for collaboration.

Causes, complexity and process of categorising 'impairment'

Introduction

This chapter begins by examining the distribution of those impairments which are commonly found in disabled people. It looks at some of the causes of these impairments. Injuries and illnesses are not evenly distributed through populations, but rather cluster around particular social groups. Second, it identifies some boundary cases of impairments whose status as a 'disability' is contested. Third, it outlines some of the complex variations in people with the same impairment label. Fourth, it examines some of the cultural classificatory categories for constituting and treating impairment. Finally, it makes a case for the importance of 'impairment literacy' as a way of gaining phenomenological insight into embodied experiences of disability.

By undertaking a review of impairment, I do not mean to follow the common-sense assumption that impairments cause disability. Impairments are *universal*, an intrinsic part of the human condition, yet only some impaired people are disabled. Social model theorists would argue that impairment has no more relevance to the topic of disability than the study of sex organs has to the study of gender, or the study of skin colour has to the study of 'race'. Furthermore, in its attempt to foster pride in difference, the disabled people's movement places a positive value on certain 'impairments'. To examine the causes or complex nature of impairment may be seen as implying a return to personal tragedy theory and the assumption that the impairment is 'the problem'.

Why then, in a book about disability, should we have a chapter which examines the social causes, consequences and meanings of impairment? The answer to this question is that disability emerges from a complex constellation of social, physiological and psychological factors. To leave out impairment means that it becomes difficult to distinguish disability from other forms of oppression.

The numbers game

I shall begin by examining some official statistics that identify the extent and causes of impairments common to disabled people. However, a word of caution is needed here. Official statistics are usually compiled in order to distribute benefits and plan services. As such, they rely upon data deemed relevant to their own objectives, and this data may not reflect fully the complex experiences of disability within a population. Assessment of the incidence of impairment is shaped in part by the definitions and practices of enumeration deployed. Thus, the assumption of the possibility of unproblematic measurement of impairment is open to challenge.

For now, I will identify some of the key statistics on impairment and disability. For the world as a whole, it has been claimed that 10 per cent of the population (an estimated 500 million people globally) has a serious impairment. In the USA, estimates of the prevalence of disability range from 35 million to as high as 43 million (Shapiro, 1994). In the UK, according to the latest official government figures, there are 8.6 million disabled people (Benn, 1998). Disabled people make up the largest minority group in many countries.

The global distribution of impairments identified by UNESCO estimates that mobility impairments are the largest category (32 per cent), followed by severe intellectual impairment (26 per cent), hearing impairment (14 per cent), epilepsy (13 per cent) and, finally, visual impairment (11 per cent). The causes of impairment are broken down in the following way: malnutrition (20 per cent), congenital diseases (20 per cent) and non-infectious diseases (20 per cent), followed by accident, trauma or war (15.6 per cent) and 'other', including ageing (13.2 per cent) (Bowron, 1998).

However, statistical information on the incidence of impairment is far from objective. Many governments have not carried out the necessary research to make an accurate assessment. In any event, what comes to be defined as disability and impairment varies greatly depending on cultures and circumstances within particular countries. For example, Shapiro (1994) points out that the US figures often do not include those with learning disabilities, mental illness and AIDS or HIV. Second, the figure of ten per cent is largely based on research carried out in wealthier countries where people live longer and where the majority of disabled people are elderly. In Africa many disabled people do not survive long enough to be included in statistics.

(Bowron, 1998)

Despite such difficulties in identifying aetiology and the extent of serious impairments on a global level, a review of statistics does have some value. For example, it can demonstrate the roles which class and demographics play in the distribution of particular kinds of impairments.

Causes of serious impairments

Development, poverty and impairment

During the late stages of the Industrial Revolution in the West, the conditions of factory production produced high levels of disablement among the working classes. Engels, in *The Condition of the Working Class in England*, commented that 'it is easy to identify such cripples at a glance, because their deformities are all exactly the same. They are knock-kneed and deformed and the spinal column is bent either forwards or sideways' (Engels, 1958: 173).

Poverty was, and still is an important factor in the distribution of impairment and disability. Poor people are more likely to be injured as a result of unsafe working conditions, wars, poor housing and poor sanitation. In those parts of the developing world which suffer from high levels of malnutrition, infectious diseases and low levels of access to immunisation and health care, levels of impairment are high. Eighty per cent of disabled people live in the developing world and 90 per cent of this group live in rural areas; many of them have been left behind in rural regions following urbanisation (Bowron, 1998).

Violence

Self-harm and attacks by others, whether in domestic settings or public arenas, is a major cause of impairment. Murphy (1987) shows that the chief cause of paraplegia and quadriplegia in US cities are gunshot wounds, which disproportionately affect those living in poor African-American neighbourhoods. War produces particular constellations of impairment. The unprecedented scale and severity of mutilations produced by artillery fire, combined with insanitary conditions on the front line and lack of antibiotics in the First World War, led to 'amputations on a scale never seen before, or since' (Bourke, 1996: 33). Such 'dismemberment was beyond the imagination of many civilians in Britain' (1996: 34). Whilst impairment was a fact of life for civilian communities prior to the First World War, this was primarily in the population of older or sick people, rather than amongst fit young conscripted men. More recent national and international conflicts have also greatly affected civilians. For example, in recent years, up to 95,000 civilians have been disabled by landmines in Angola and Mozambique (Bowron, 1998).

Chronic and acute illness and injury

In the nineteenth century, the leading causes of impairment and death in the USA and the UK were acute illnesses and accidents. These included the effects of pneumonia, tuberculosis, gastro-enteritis and a range of injuries. The medical system is now well-equipped to deal with such acute and traumatic illnesses and injuries. Take spinal cord injury as an example. In the First World War, 90 per cent of men with wounds that paralysed their lower bodies died before they reached home. By the later 1960s, 85 per cent of those paralysed during the Second World War were still alive (Shapiro, 1994). Today, complications for people with spinal cord injuries, such as respiratory problems and bladder infections which once killed, can be routinely dealt with and quadriplegics can live long lives. Thus 'gains in lives saved by advances in the care of injury victims have contributed to the prevalence of disabling conditions in the United States' (Pope and Tarlov, 1991: 147). Shapiro documents some of the medical treatments which have helped people to survive with serious impairments.

> in the mid-1970's, 90 per cent of people with severe head injuries died; today 90 per cent live. Premature babies born at twenty-three or twenty-four weeks old, instead of the usual forty weeks, live now too. ... Today, almost 50 per cent weighing as little as one pound, two ounces, to one pound, ten ounces, survive, and the majority will have some disabling neurological condition.
>
> (Shapiro, 1994: 6)

Thus, medicine has increased the number of survivors from injuries to the spinal cord and brain.

In contrast to the nineteenth century, the fastest growing segment of the British and US populations is made up of those over the age of 65, and the main causes of illness and impairment are long-term – chronic diseases of the heart, cancers, vascular lesions of the central nervous system and diabetes. These modern conditions tend to be associated with ageing rather than contagion and the vast majority of impairments are now acquired rather than congenital.

Environment, lifestyle and health

Another major factor contributing to changes in the level and type of impairment has been the changing environment. By this I refer not just to the physical environment (although this has seen ecological damage caused by pollutants which have been correlated with a rise in chronic respiratory disease such as asthma) but also to lifestyle changes such as the availability of fast foods and sedentary habits leading to a rise in obesity and other impairments or illnesses. Alongside these problems there has been a rise in illnesses which are seen as stress-related. As Turner writes, 'stress has replaced the germ as the major explanation of modern illness; the concept of cures will be increasingly replaced by concepts of rehabilitation and care' (Turner, 1995: 8).

The picture of impairments and chronic illnesses caused by diet, ecology and the organisation of work is constantly changing. For example, after thirty years of rising rates of coronary heart disease in the USA, a reduction in smoking and in the levels of saturated fat eaten has led to a reduction in deaths due to heart attacks. Similarly, greater safety features built into cars and the compulsory wearing of seat belts in the UK have produced a reduction in serious injuries from road accidents.

Accommodating 'differences': judgements about responsibility

In reviewing the official statistics about the extent and nature of impairments, I have implied that impairments are relatively fixed and non-controversial 'facts' of life. By contrast, disability is socially produced and reproduced because of the way impairments are perceived and treated. Later, I shall argue that whilst this distinction

– made by social model theorists – between disability and impairment serves a useful pragmatic function, it does not stand up to analytic scrutiny.

For now it is important to make the point that even if we accept the dualistic model of impairment and disability propounded by social model theorists, what comes to be identified as disabled (in other words, what the social consequences of impairments are) in contemporary advanced Western culture is highly contested. When we accept a person into the category 'disabled' we may be entitling them to certain benefits or subjecting them to an oppressive label. When new legislation and new benefits providing goods, services or protection for disabled people are introduced, then official definitions of disability change. New groups of people 'become' disabled. This is not to imply that such people are frauds, but rather to show the extent to which disability is an administrative concept.

Examples of some particularly contested questions are whether 'invisible' impairments, such as mental illness, and aesthetic impairments, such as facial 'disfigurement', should be treated as disabilities. If so, should the UK government pay for cosmetic surgery when the applicant claims that their appearance is causing them mental health problems? Should airlines provide twice as much seating area for a clinically 'obese' person who cannot fit into one seat? Should employers accept responsibility and pay compensation to an employee who has developed repetitive strain injury? Should accommodations be made for the pupil who has difficulties concentrating in class, and whose parents claim he (it usually is a boy) has attention deficit disorder? Should the rules of a sport be adapted so everyone can participate (e.g. should the rules requiring golfers to walk be relaxed for those whose impairment makes walking difficult)? Should the authorities offer compensation to someone who, after witnessing a human disaster, suffers from recurring flashbacks and lapses in concentration?

In other words, does the attempt to create a level playing field for all individual differences take away individual responsibility? Further, does it rely on the fantasy that social rules can be both meaningful and endlessly flexible? To what extent can science, politics, economics or ethics answer these questions? Where do we draw the line between the attempt to create an environment that accommodates everyone perfectly and an environment that is exclusive, rigid and unfairly discriminatory? These medical model/moral definitional wrangles are not solely the preserve of the state and large institutions with vested interests in exclusionary practices. They also make up an important feature of contemporary socio-cultural discussions about what the 'norm' should be and to what extent differences are tolerated.

All of these examples (you may well be able to think of other recent highly publicised cases) show how 'disability' is not easily established, but is constituted through negotiations between people in different institutional and hierarchical contexts. The concept of disability is not just an administrative idea or an economic category, produced in order to determine the distribution of benefits and services. It is also a moral concept, related to perceptions of responsibility. Whether someone is defined as disabled or not depends in part on our understanding of who is responsible for their impairments and whether they have a moral right to expect assistance and accommodation in their different needs. The state deals with these questions as a matter of establishing citizenship rights. Later on in the chapter, some of the moral values implicit in classifications of disability will be examined.

Perceiving impairment

When we look more closely at who is included in contemporary statistics, we appreciate the complex tasks involved in policing the boundaries between disabled and non-disabled people. One assumption of many non-disabled people is that impairments are always visible. Yet many disabled people are not readily identified as such. For example, people with a heart condition or mental illness may look perfectly 'able', and many people may have impairments which are only occasionally visible. The person with epilepsy, for example, will be aware of the risk of having a seizure. They may be on anti-convulsant drugs which have powerful side effects. They may be refused a driving licence and discriminated against in a job application if they 'come out' about their epilepsy. One important factor which distinguishes an invisible, or more accurately, an imperceptible impairment, is that a person has some control over the extent to which others are informed about it.

Goffman (1963) identifies those who have characteristics which are both stigmatised and invisible as 'discreditable'. Such a person is faced with a dilemma of whether or not to display their impairment. Goffman distinguishes the perceptibility of a stigma from three other notions which are often confused with it.

First, the visibility of a stigma must be distinguished from its 'known-about-ness'. ... Secondly, visibility must be distinguished from its ... obtrusiveness. When a stigma is immediately perceivable, the issue still remains as to how much it interferes with the flow of interaction. ... Thirdly, the visibility of a stigma ... must be disentangled from certain possibilities of what can be called its 'perceived focus'. ... Ugliness, for example [may] ... threaten the pleasure we might otherwise take in the company of its possessor. We perceive, however, that his condition ought to have no effect on his competency in solitary tasks.

(Goffman, 1963: 65–7)

Goffman makes great play of the politics of perception or 'impression management' in the construction of disability. Because impairments are not always perceptible, and only some impairments become disabling, it becomes much harder to identify who 'the disabled' are. It is not possible to understand the physical, intellectual or emotional condition of a person from looking at them.

Degrees or levels of impairment

Uncertainty about how to categorise people is crucially significant in raising anxiety among many non-disabled people in their dealings with disabled people. The whole question of categorising 'others' lies at the heart of a number of issues related to the definition of disability, the organisation of disability politics, the administration of benefits and the treatment of disabled people.

We tend to deploy medical categories as if they were clear-cut and straightforward. We have all seen movies in which the doctor, after examining the patient, breaks the news to a relative that the patient will 'never walk again' or has 'six months to live'. This suggests a degree of certainty about the nature of a condition which is afforded by a short diagnostic label. Such faith in the diagnostic accuracy of doctors has led to parents of impaired newborn babies being told to 'expect nothing' or prepare themselves for an early death. When Jane Campbell was born in 1959, the doctors told her mother to

take her home and enjoy her while she lived – they predicted a life of about a year at the most. As is often the case where named conditions are concerned, they got it wrong, and she is very much alive, chairing the BCODP, which is the national (UK) representative voice of the disability movement.

(Campbell and Oliver, 1996: 3)

The next section of this chapter examines three broad types of physical impairment and looks at the wide range of differences between people categorised within them. Such an analysis has an important educative function in that it shows the dangers of making assumptions about the experiences of impairment. Disabilities, just like abilities, occur on a continuum and it is just as unhelpful to put all disabled people in the same category as it is to classify all able bodied people as one.

Of the one million people in the UK who are registered as blind or partially sighted, only 4 per cent have no sight at all and 14 per cent have light perception only. The rest have enough vision to cope with many aspects of life, although within the group of partially sighted people there are huge differences in the nature and extent of impairment. In addition, the nature of visual impairment can differ dramatically. Some people who are blind or have severe visual impairments are, for example, able to see long distances despite having little peripheral vision.

Yet such variability is not generally well understood. Sally French writes of adults who, when she was a child, tended to

> disbelieve me and interpret my behaviour as 'playing up' when I told them I could not see. Basically they were confused and unable to cope with the ambiguities of partial sight and were not prepared to take instruction on the matter from a mere child. ... On several occasions I was told off by opticians when I failed to discriminate between the different lenses they placed before my eyes. I am not sure whether they really disbelieved me or whether their professional pride was hurt when nothing they could offer seemed to help; whatever it was I rapidly learned to say 'better' or 'worse', even though all the lenses looked the same.
>
> (French; 1994: 69–70)

The question of the authenticity of people's accounts dominates many representations of disability. As in the case of visual impairments, most people who are registered deaf have some residual hearing. Of the 7.5 million people with hearing difficulties, three-quarters are over 60 years old. '[P]relingually deaf persons form a relatively small proportion of the estimated 7.5 million people with some loss of hearing' (Lysons, 1996: x). Of the total adult population 11.33 per cent experience mild hearing loss, whilst only 0.54 per cent of the population have severe hearing loss, and only 0.14 per cent of the population have profound hearing loss (figures from Lysons, 1996: xi). Some hard of hearing and deaf people will be able to hear more through the use of a hearing aid of which there are a wide range of different types. Such a range is necessary because there are wide variations not just in the degree of hearing loss, but also in the nature of that loss. Some people's ability to discriminate sounds is greatly impaired, whilst others have greatest difficulties with sounds at the high or low end of the decibel range. Conversely, those with conductive hearing loss, arising from damage to the outer or middle ear, can hear their own voice through bone conduction, and can tolerate loud sounds and speech. Those with sensorineural loss arising in the inner ear and beyond (the cochlea or nerve pathways) may have difficulty hearing their own voice and may find loud sounds painful. Finally, some forms of hearing loss may involve abnormalities affecting both the conductive and sensorineural mechanisms.

In the case of mobility impairments, there is a great deal of similar misunderstanding about the possible range of functioning. People with little experience of spinal cord injury, for example, may refer to someone being paralysed 'from the waist down'. However, this description of paraplegia belies the wide range of effects which different forms of spinal injury may have. Hockenberry (1996) writes,

'Paralyzed from the waist down' describes so little of the experiences of a spinal-cord injury that most crips use it as a kind of shorthand joke. In my case I am paralyzed from the nipples down. When people learn of this they are shocked to realise that there is no international checkpoint at the waist. It is an arbitrary demarcation. In actual fact, relatively few people are paralyzed from the waist down. Everyone has their particular line separating sensation from numbness. Each line of separation is invisible to the eye. In some people the aspects of temperature and pressure and muscle control are separate. Some spinal-cord-injured people can feel pressure but not temperature in some parts of their body, and vice versa. There are people with almost total sensation but with no motor control ... a partially damaged fiber-optic cable ... picture but no sound ... bad reception. All these metaphors aid understanding, but none is precise. The trace of each paraplegic and quadriplegic's sensory border zone is as unique as a fingerprint. Each person has a different answer to the question: What does paralysis feel like?.

(Hockenberry, 1996: 97)

Later on, Hockenberry goes on to address an issue that evokes a great deal of curiosity about the degree of control which spinal cord injured people have over sexual and elimination functions.

Lower injuries between the base and the middle of the spine generally mean that while the body retains more muscle control, more use of legs and abdominals, it is incontinent, impotent and incapable of having an orgasm. Injuries above the middle mean more severe paralysis in terms of pure muscle loss, but because the voluntary and involuntary nerves can talk to each other on what's left of the spinal cord, bladders stay closed and an orgasm is possible if difficult. The effect of the curious neural ordering is to divide the wheelchair crips (males particularly) into jocks and sex gods.

(Hockenberry, 1996: 100)

This complex picture of the variations and degree of impairment in deafness, blindness and spinal cord injury is unfamiliar to many non-disabled people, who do not have personal experience of such impairments. Most people in our contemporary segregated society have to rely on melodramatic media. They rely on literary images of blindness as 'total darkness', deafness as 'total silence' and spinal cord injury as 'total paralysis' (which, however, can be mystically overcome with 'enough determination'). All these images function to constitute the states of 'ability' and 'disability' as radically different, rather than as part of a wide and complex human spectrum.

Stability of impairments

As with the question of the variability across a range, which is simplified into binary categories, the states of ability and disability, and illness and health are often seen as fixed and stable within a particular individual. However, one aspect shared by all humans, whatever their physiological condition, is that these boundaries may be crossed. Foucault writes, in *The Archaeology of Knowledge*, 'don't ask me who I am and don't ask me to remain the same'. Although Foucault was talking about the discursive construction of identity, his statement may also apply to our unstable physical and emotional states, which are in a constant state of flux.

However, the kinds of struggles experienced by those with chronic or degenerative illnesses, such as multiple sclerosis, Parkinson's disease and ME, produce more dramatic changes in their physical, emotional or intellectual functioning. This is particularly the case for those suffering from 'mental illness' or emotional distress. Periods of breakdown, depression or anxiety may be interspersed with periods of greater emotional stability and contentment. People with epilepsy or asthma may go through periods that are relatively free from seizures or breathing difficulties. As a consequence of this, disabled people may experience greater or lesser levels of 'disability' at different times in their lives or even different moments in the day. Zola (1988) has pointed out that:

> While we do, of course, recognise that some diseases are progres-sive, we are less inclined to see that there is no one-time, overall adaptation or adjustment to the condition, no set treatment, and most important, no set design requirement for an individual's working and living situations. Even for a recognised progressive and episodic disorder such as multiple sclerosis, only recently has attention been given to the continuous nature of adaptations.
>
> (Zola, 1988: 366)

This point raises the importance of the question of the life stages of the ill or disabled person. Whilst the social model shows that some impairments become important only in certain social environments, impairments also have different social implications according to the age of a person. For example, 'sexual and reproductive issues are less important for the very young and the very old, and some for only one sex' (Zola, 1988: 369)[1]. The changes in the nature of impair-ments produce different medical effects for people of different ages, as Zola demonstrates in the following example:

> With the survival into adulthood of people with diseases that once were usually fatal, comes changes and complications.

Problems of circulation and vision for people with diabetes, for example, may be due to the disease itself, to the ageing process, or even to the life-sustaining treatment.

(Zola, 1988: 368)

What this discussion of variation in the visibility, degree and stability of impairments shows is that the experience of impairment is highly variable between individuals. Not only is 'ability' contingent (as discussed in Chapter 1), but degree of impairment is also subject to fluctuation.

The cultural importance of classification

Having argued that impairments are variable in different people and across time, it is interesting to explore how different cultures deal with those people who are constituted as abnormal. More specifically, why are people with particular impairments deemed not merely abnormal, but also potentially contaminating to those constituted as 'able'? This question is explored in a paper by Murphy *et al.* (1988). Before outlining their argument, it is helpful to summarise the anthropological ideas of Douglas (1991 [1966]) which lie at the heart of Murphy *et al.*'s argument.

Douglas argues that there is nothing objective about what comes to be seen as dirt or cleanliness, food or non-food. Rather, uncleanness is simply 'matter out of place, we must approach it through order. Uncleanness or dirt is that which must not be included if a pattern is to be maintained' (1991 [1966]: 41). In other words, anomalies arising from a system of classification become taboo. All cultures engage in arbitrary classification of matter: for example, what is considered food, and how and when it is eaten. Thus, for Jewish people, there are rules about which animals may be eaten, how they are killed and how meat should be separated from dairy products. Precisely because the distinctions between categories are relatively arbitrary, they generate exceptions and 'boundary cases'. Thus, 'any given system of classification must give rise to anomalies, and any given culture must confront events which seem to defy its assumptions' (Douglas, 1991 [1966]: 40). This is particularly the case for matter or phenomena which exist at the 'margins' of a category, such as spit or faeces, which lie at the boundary of the human body, emerging from inside yet are also separate from the body. This type of matter is constituted as contaminating and is kept apart from ideal classifications through a range of taboos which function to protect the purity of the symbolic order. Anomalies may also be dealt with by generating a new category in order to give a symbolic location to the anomaly. Physical power may be exerted in order to remove an anomaly. For example, night-crowing cocks are killed in some societies so 'they do not live to contradict the definition of a cock as a bird that crows at dawn' (Douglas, 1991 [1966]: 40).

Douglas gives the example, drawn from Evans-Pritchard's ethnography, of the Nuer, who 'treat monstrous births [sic] as baby hippopotamuses, accidentally born to humans and, with this labelling, the appropriate action is clear. They gently lay them in the river where they belong' (Douglas, 1991 [1966]: 40). This move by the Nuer to generate the new non-human category of 'baby hippopotamus' when presented with an anomalous baby, is particularly instructive when thinking about the classification and treatment of disabled people. Such agreement to define certain anomalous births as 'monstrous' and non-human is, as discussed in Chapter 2, one strategy that certain utilitarian philosophers have used in their discussions of what constitutes a life worth living.

Finally, Douglas suggests that rituals can function 'to unify' anomalies (1991 [1966]: 40–1) by establishing a grand pattern which reincorporates that which is constituted as matter out of place. Douglas draws upon Van Gennep's concept of liminality in order to develop this exploration of the function of ritual in maintaining classificatory systems. Liminality describes the position of those people who are difficult to locate within social categories. When a person is in a liminal condition, they are temporarily without firm identity or role definition:

> they have died in their old status and are not reborn in a new one. In a very real sense, they are non persons, making all interaction with them unpredictable and problematic ... the liminal are socially dangerous people, and the solution is to sequester them, interacting with them only within the protective armour provided by ritual formalism.
>
> (Murphy, 1987: 237)

Liminality thus refers to the state which is encountered during a stage in life when a person enters an undefined and socially ambivalent status. Such a stage is often marked by rites of passage that ritualise separation and transition through stages. Confirmations and bar mitzvahs offer Western examples of such life-stage rituals for those who are between childhood and adulthood, involving separation and instruction. Murphy *et al.* argue that much rehabilitation training involves withdrawal from mainstream culture in order to learn how to live in one's new status. Like the sick role, which condones suspension from social obligations, rehabilitation training offers a 'liminal' space prior to the development of a new disabled identity.

Disability becomes a taboo subject because, according to Murphy *et al.*, it represents phenomena which do not fit into the current social and symbolic order, 'and the non-disabled commonly deal with this indefinition in the same way in which most ambivalent relations are handled by setting up social distance through either hyperbole of conduct or avoidance' (Murphy *et al.*, 1988: 238).

The concept of liminality seems to have some relevance for making sense of the anxiety felt around some disabled people whose impairments are not understood. It is a concept which is particularly helpful in making sense of what Goffman (1963) describes as 'sticky interactions' between 'normals' and the 'stigmatised'. Anxiety is born of uncertainty regarding how to interact with, and fear of contamination from, those constituted as 'neither sick nor well, neither fully alive nor quite dead' (Murphy *et al.*, 1988: 238). The social uncertainty felt by 'normals' when interacting with those people who have been structurally segregated from mainstream spaces is intensified when interacting with those disabled people who have difficulty managing their movements and controlling their bodily products. Murphy gives the example of 'a hemiplegic or a person with cerebral palsy [who] may have trouble controlling saliva' (1988: 239), and thus may generate anxiety in a culture which emphasises the importance of keeping bodily products either inside the body or removed from sight. An adult who dribbles thus violates strict cultural codes regarding bodily management and self-regulation[2].

Embodiment

Elias in his study of the civilising process, *The History of Manners* (1978), shows that bodies have not always been subject to strict control. In medieval times, there was much weaker demarcation between the social and natural environment, and fewer prohibitions were placed on the public display of bodily functioning. For example, defecating in the streets was common. From the Renaissance onwards, Western European countries instigated a series of codes relating to etiquette, which involved socialising bodies so that they became the location for the expression of behavioural codes that were used to reflect social hierarchy and court value systems (Elias, 1983). Natural bodily rhythms were hidden away and bodies increasingly came to be used as markers for identity and value. Elias' discussion of the civilising process adds an embodied phenomenological dimension to the cultural analysis offered by Goffman and by Murphy *et al.* To develop this focus on the body as the material location for symbolic interactions, it is useful to turn to the work of phenomenologists such as Bourdieu, and disability theorists such as Patterson, who have addressed the question of embodiment in relation to disability.

Before examining Bourdieu's notion of 'habitus' and its relevance to understanding disabling interactions, it is important to outline the meaning of the term 'embodiment', which presents a significant challenge to the Cartesian mind/body dualism discussed in Chapter 3. The concept of embodiment grounds perception not in a mind – as a fundamentally different substance from the material body – but in the *intentional experiencing* body. Merleau-Ponty (1962) sees the body as an active creator of significance and the site of meaningful expression. The body should not be seen as matter set apart from subjectivity and the environment, but as an entity inextricably bound up with creative meaning and context. Bourdieu examines the way in which the body adopts a particular habitual way of relating to the environment. The ways in which we deport ourselves and manage interactions in a specific familiar social and material environment are part of what Bourdieu refers to as 'habitus'. This habitus emerges through experiences which shape the stance we adopt in the world. As Bourdieu puts it,

> To speak of habitus is to assert that the individual, and even the personal, the subjective, is social, collective. Habitus is a socialised subjectivity ... neither the individual ... nor groups as concrete sets of individuals sharing a similar location in social space, but in relation between two realisations of historical action, in bodies and in things.
>
> (Bourdieu, 1992: 126)

> Habitus ... is an *open system of dispositions* that is constantly subjected to experiences, and therefore constantly affected by them in a way that either reinforces or modifies its structures.
>
> (Bourdieu, 1992: 133)

Merleau-Ponty and Bourdieu offer different ways of investigating the lived experiences of corporeal 'embodied' people. Such interest in embodiment has become a key concern amongst social researchers wishing to bring a new material dimension to the notion of the 'personal as political'. Researchers into the sociology of health and illness have examined the range of ways in which the body is both active and acted upon. For example, the sociological work on pain emphasises that pain cannot be understood as merely a physiological effect. It always has meaning; it is always 'socially informed' (Csordas, 1993: 3), and can only therefore be understood in terms of the specific location of a person in space and time (Bendelow and Williams, 1995). Crossley (1995) suggests that we need to look at the way values, conventional practices, time and space are 'carnally informed'.

According to Patterson (1998), a 'carnal sociology of the body' can be used to examine the embodied experiences of impairment. This opens up an important new dimension to our understanding of the oppression of disabled people. Patterson takes Goffman's notion of 'shared vocabularies of body idiom' to show how temporal and spatial conventions of interaction exclude people with communication impairments. He writes:

> codes of movement and timing are based on a carnal order which is informed primarily by non-impaired bodies. ... The scripts for communication, timing and proprioception are therefore pre-disposed to the exclusion of people with impairments. It is not the exclusion from social space (which has been the central concern of the social model of disability) which is at issue here, but ostracism from opportunities to participate in the everyday, mundane, sensate minutiae of the lifeworld.
>
> (Patterson, 1998: 71)

Patterson (1998) and Patterson and Hughes (1997) draw usefully on phenomenology to bring a new embodied critical understanding of disability. They demonstrate the importance of fostering greater understanding of the way certain impaired people are excluded from social interaction. One evocative example of the way 'the carnal order is informed' by sighted bodies is given by Hull:

> When somebody turns the juke-box on in the coffee bar, the sound literally obliterates the voices of my friends. It is as if I was alone. They disappear. Only the juke-box exists. ... This is why I find noisy parties, especially discos, so lonely. People have to tap me on the shoulder to attract my attention. It is like having headphones on and not being able to take them off.
>
> (Hull, 1997: 152)

Having argued in Chapter 4 that social structures shape disability, in this chapter I have examined bodily differences and practices shaping the form of disablism. This raises the question of the extent to which education can help people develop a more inclusive way of carnally relating to a wider range of people. What form might education about impairment take? To what extent can a critical insight into the experience of impairment assist people to transform disabling cultural classifications and disabling embodied practices?

Impairment literacy[3]

Impairment literacy involves some knowledge of the nature and consequence of particular forms of impairment. Those people who are close to someone disabled are more likely to be more sensitive and educated about that person's particular impairment. However, since disabled people have been isolated and segregated from mainstream society, many non-disabled people have been deprived of contact with disabled people, and therefore of the opportunity of learning about particular impairments. Such widespread ignorance creates practical difficulties for many disabled people in gaining appropriate assistance and, more generally, in feeling understood. John Hull captures something of this problem in his autobiography which describes his experience of becoming blind. In the first extract, Hull describes his happy experience at a meeting of 'an association for the blind':

> It was curious and in a strange way rather comforting to find myself in a situation where the little habits which characterise the response of blind people to the world were accepted by a social group. The meeting began, for example, by everybody

announcing who was present. This sometimes takes place in a sighted group when there is about to be a discussion, but I have never known it at the start of a business meeting. In the social exchange after the business meeting, there was a tremendous hubbub. People were simply shouting out the names of those they wanted to speak with, and in reply, you simply forced your way through the crowd towards whoever was shouting out your name.

(Hull, 1997: 150)

Compare this happy description with the awkward and frustrating experience in this second extract, in which Hull is talking to a sighted woman at a residential conference:

As we walked across the crowded lounge, I said to her brightly, 'you know, I have to train people the way they train guide dogs for the blind. I have a special technique for people to sit me down in an armchair. Would you like me to train you in it?' Laughingly, she agreed. 'OK,' I said. 'This is what we do. When we get to the chair, you take one of my hands, stretch it out, and place it on the back of the chair.' When we got to the chair she couldn't do this. Maybe the lounge chair was in an awkward position or something. I suggested that she should put her own hand on the back of the chair. She did this, by now thoroughly mystified. I simply ran my fingers along her arm and located the back of the chair. Immediately, I was orientated. I needed no further help. I knew exactly where the chair was, and I could now sit down any time I liked, with safety and dignity. My companion, however, refused to let go. 'Thank you,' I said cheerfully. 'That was very good. You can let go now and I will sit down.' She was determined to back me into the chair, holding both my elbows from the front. After a few more appeals I persuaded her to let go and I sat down.

(Hull, 1997: 100)

Disabled people are frequently compelled to go through the task of 'training' people who are unfamiliar with 'people like them'. This training can be excruciating, as the account given by Hull demonstrates. Perhaps the non-disabled woman became so anxious about what to do, that her capacity to listen to John Hull became impaired (see Bion, 1961, for an account of the effects of anxiety on the capacity to think). Perhaps she resented being subjected to a 'training session' rather than a simple request for assistance. Perhaps she arrogantly thought she knew best, and didn't trust Hull's capacity to sit, even when he insisted he had oriented himself.

When interacting with people with communication difficulties, non-disabled people often panic about unfamiliar ways of speaking, and therefore are unable to 'hear' what is being said. Both the responses of adopting a colonising stance of certainty or of panicking may represent the fear of appearing stupid, of not knowing what to do. Arrogance and helplessness may represent two sides of the same coin. However, the effect of failing to engage with the disabled person may be the same.

Sometimes, even when the non-disabled person is sensitive, respectful and politically aware, their unfamiliarity with a particular impairment can impede successful communication or facilitative responses. For example, the concern within the disabled people's movement to ensure that disabled people have greater choices and control over their lives is a central part of campaigning. Yet presenting choices to autistic people who have been placed within the category of having a learning disability may be experienced as bewildering and even threatening. A person who is autistic often needs the security of routines in order to feel safe (Williams, 1994; Tustin, 1992). Being 'empowered' with choices may, for an autistic person, be experienced as a shattering of security.

If it is accepted that a certain degree of impairment literacy is useful in challenging the tyranny of disabling environments and ablist embodied knowledge and practices, then consideration needs to be given regarding the form that education might take.

Disability equality training

The disabled people's movement has been very critical of approaches which focus on education about impairment. Attempts to educate non-disabled people about the physical consequences of impairment are seen as reproducing an individual orientation. In preference to such an approach, many disability equality trainers or consultants favour educating people about disabling environments. It is possible to make the analogy of such a focus on equality with anti-racist training, since both concentrate on the socio-political context that discriminates against racialised or disabled 'others'. However, just as anti-racist training can be enriched by multi-culturalism, so education about the politics of disablement can be supplemented with some basic education regarding the nature and consequences of impairments.

Impairment simulation

Despite the value of demystifying impairments, it is important to add a cautionary note regarding certain forms of 'awareness training' and, in particular, 'disability simulation'. Simulation exercises attempt to give non-disabled people an insight into the experience of impairment. This might be done by getting shop assistants to use wheelchairs, attach weights to their arms or wear blindfolds in training sessions in order to increase their appreciation of barriers to shopping. However, such training often fails to capture some of the most difficult aspects of their impairment, such as the effect of cumulative frustration, pain, fatigue or social isolation. On the other hand, simulation can also over-estimate some aspects of difficulties. People using a wheelchair for the first time will not have built up their upper body strength or gained the proficiency achieved by a seasoned wheelchair user. Rather than listening to what disabled people are saying, simulation may pander to voyeuristic excitement and give non-disabled people the opportunity to colonise the experience of disability. Simulation may lead to, at best, a very distorted and reductive kind of 'empathy', a cavalier fantasy that an experience has been understood, or an increase in pity for the disabled person.

It is salient, therefore, to ask if there are any instances in which simulation can be empowering rather than oppressive? The answer to this question is that it depends who controls the exercises and whether they are introduced in a way that contextualises the experience. Impairment simulation is less likely to lead to reductive assumptions if training is undertaken by disabled people, who are put in the position of the expert rather than the 'object' of curiosity and concern. Fostering empathy is not, on its own, an effective strategy for challenging disablist assumptions. It must be combined with education about disabling environments. Allowing a person to experience use of a wheelchair could therefore be combined with a trip around real disabling environments in order to learn about the specific nature of physical barriers[4]. In this way, training may foster complex embodied knowledge of barriers as well as an awareness of the limits of these barriers.

Permission to explore fears and fantasies

Having identified ways of training people in order to foster embodied empathy regarding disablism, it remains to explore how training may also address some of the unconscious anxieties associated with disability. Disability and Dedication (DAD) is a small voluntary group of disabled people in Sheffield, most of whom are wheelchair users, who are engaged in educating children about disability. They go into schools, where, after a short presentation, 'the team circulates a map of an ordinary room highlighting obstacles and difficulties presented to a disabled person'. They offer to answer any question (including 'rude' ones) which the children have. They write in their brochure,

> young people can be disarmingly and refreshingly honest. ... For example, the children in Year 7 ... wanted to know if Paul felt depressed or angry, how he ate, how he washed, who would care for him if he didn't have a family, how his children felt about it – a barrage of questions which few people would be prepared to face. Yet the team is willing to cast aside the conventions of adult conversation and answer the questions in the spirit in which they were asked.
>
> (Hattersley *et al.*, 1992)

Normally it would be intrusive to ask disabled people such intimate questions. The permission which DAD gives children to examine the validity of any fantasies they might have, sit in a wheelchair and engage in a relaxed way with speakers creates a new sense of comfort and connection between the children and disabled people generally. As Partridge (1990) shows, permission to explore differences can be an important source of education. It is crucially important that impairment literacy is developed in a context which is controlled by disabled people, so that learning does not degenerate into voyeurism. Thus, for the child who has internalised disablist values which suggest that there is something frightening or unbearable about certain kinds of differences, DAD shows that the 'unmentionable' can be discussed in an entertaining way. In some ways, the work of DAD counters the fears and fantasies engendered when children are told in hushed tones that there is something terribly unfortunate about a person, which means you should 'look away'.

In conclusion, disability equality training may be comprised of a mix of exploration of the environment, impairment and interpersonal relationships of disabled people. Ultimately, awareness training is not about understanding 'other people', but about developing the sensitivity of a range of differences in particular contexts. Given that the average person living to the age of 75 will spend 13 of these years with some limited capacity (Pope and Tarlov, 1991), such education will prepare non-disabled/contingently able-bodied people for the future.

Summary

Whilst this book does not aim to examine the physiology of impairments, this chapter has suggested that some appreciation of the complexity and variability of embodied differences may offer a valuable dimension to disability equality training. We might wish to call this 'impairment literacy'. Most adults, in contemporary Western society, whatever their disability status, have attended segregated schools (since mainstream schools involve the systematic exclusion of disabled people), and have not had the opportunity of coming into contact with a cross-section of the people. As such, when confronted with differences, responses to those constituted as 'other' can include prurience, intrusiveness, avoidance, hostility, lack of consideration and insensitivity. Impairment literacy is clearly no more the answer to disablism than multi-cultural education is to the problem of racism. However, it does help build new links between groups of people. It presents an opportunity to deal with some of the fears and fantasies around disability.

7

Does language disable people?

Introduction

This chapter looks at the way language is used to separate disabled people from 'normal' society, and to characterise the experiences of disabled people as being different and separate from the rest of society. It argues that language plays an important role in removing disability from mundane human experience, and treating it as radically 'Other'. Impairment comes to be treated as a 'master status', standing for the disabled person, who is constituted as 'not quite human' (Goffman, 1963: 15).

The chapter begins by exploring the significance of language for defining and understanding the experience of disability. It does this by outlining two key ways of interrogating language, first by examining the ways in which language is used rhetorically – how particular speech 'acts' oppress or empower disabled people – and second by examining the way in which language structures reality. In short, to what extent does disablist language construct and reproduce disability?

The chapter goes on to outline two different strategies for challenging disablist language: 'positive self-naming' (abandoning offensive terms in favour of new non-pejorative terms); and 'defiant self-naming' (reclaiming offensive terminology as an act of assertion or resistance). This latter strategy is seen as being more in tune with psychoanalytic theory as developed by Sinason in her analysis of euphemism and the emotional investments that shape the politics of language.

Stigma and metaphor

Disputes about terminology are a particular concern for disabled people. Indeed, the whole problem of labelling has been discussed earlier in this book. Language is clearly important in the construction of disability. For example, the vocabulary used to identify impairments is frequently used as terms of abuse: a person who is not aware of their surroundings and fails to notice something important may be derided as 'blind', a person who fails to listen is 'deaf', while a person who fails to understand something may be taunted with the term 'retard'. Such attacks feed back into our images of disabled people. The assumption is that blind and deaf people cannot interact effectively with their surroundings and that people with learning difficulties have no capacity to understand at all. In other words, using impairments as terms of abuse generalises and exaggerates the effect they are seen as having. However, perhaps even more insidious than direct attacks and insults is the way in which disabled people are undermined by terms which make them synonymous with their impairments. Disabled people are often simply not seen. When a disabled person is referred to in terms of their technical aids, such as 'the wheelchair person', they are not accorded the subjectivity automatically conferred on non-disabled people. No one would refer to a non-disabled person, as the 'running shoes' person. The title of the long running BBC Radio 4 programme 'Does He Take Sugar?' (which ceased broadcasting in 1999) expresses the experience of many disabled people. Sontag (1991) criticises the way in which certain states (such as illnesses) are treated as metaphors for fears and fantasies which have nothing to do with the reality of particular illnesses. Similarly, disability functions as a metaphor for 'something else', rather than a mundane and unremarkable quality that is a part of the human condition.

Cultural contexts and terminology

It is important to examine the institutional and cultural context in which terms are constituted and used. For example, in the UK, the term 'impairment' is taken for granted by the disabled people's movement to refer to bodily or mental aspects of the disabled person. However, in the international context, the term 'impairment' is often considered to be more problematic. Barnes points out that 'in some languages direct translations of impairment would have profoundly negative meaning' (Barnes, 1994: 2). Similarly, whilst 'disability' is the term used in the UK to describe social barriers, the term 'handicap' has wider currency at the international level. In the UK, the term 'handicap' has been rejected by many commentators in favour of impairment because of the patronising connotations of being 'cap-in-hand'; that is, of begging.

Versions of social constructionism

Language is not a transparent referential system. It does not refer straightforwardly and objectively to objects in the external world. Since the 1970s, philosophers, sociologists and critical psychologists have shown that language plays a key role in constituting our perceptions (Hall, 1997). Indeed, as Edwards *et al.* (1995) argue, 'naive realists' (those who believe objective perception of the external world is possible) no longer exist in the social sciences except as 'straw' people. If the empirical world is shaped by the symbolic resources we have available to see that world, then social constructionism can counter the claims of those who position themselves as experts with the assertion that 'things could be different'.

There is, however, dispute among social constructionists regarding the relative importance of the systemic/structural and the functional aspects of language. In general, whilst the importance of examining the impact of language is acknowledged, there is disagreement regarding the extent to which language routinely and procedurally reproduces social inequality, and what can be done to bring about change.

Language use

The British analytical philosopher Austin (1962) argued that talk should be viewed not as a series of descriptions, but rather as action. For example, if someone says they are feeling exhausted, they may be describing an internal state, caused by lack of sleep or lots of physical exercise. However, their language also serves to achieve a particular effect (e.g. to warn their flatmate not to wake them up too early). The value of 'speech act theory', and its subsequent development by conversational analysts and ethnomethodologists (Garfinkel, 1967), is that it does not take speech claims on their own terms, but examines the way in which language functions.

Take, for example, the following statement: 'I do a lot of charity work for those confined to wheelchairs, so you can't accuse me of being against the disabled.' The speaker is projecting an image of themselves as selfless, and of the person they are helping as trapped. They are also using the self-justifying device similar to those who say 'some of my best friends' prior to attacking a particular category of person. This somewhat crude example shows that it is important to look not just at the manifest meaning of a statement, but also to examine how it functions for the self-image the speaker is attempting to project.

Another example of a rhetorical strategy commonly used to maintain a disabling status quo is the use of 'extreme case formulations' (Pomerantz, 1986) to discredit those arguing for change. For example, critics of the social model may accuse it of advocating the supply of elevators in every home – a patently unrealistic demand for a perfect environment (Marks, 1998), which few disability rights campaigners would bother making.

In addition to these examples of the way in which language is used to disguise and reproduce disablism or to discredit calls for change, language may also be used strategically to resist disablist oppression. Parents discussing their children's 'handicaps' emphasise pragmatic rather than fixed or principled use of terminology. Ablon offers the following examples from interviews.

> Lisa has no vision of herself as handicapped. But we would have no problem using the term handicapped if we need to get her anything. It wouldn't bother her or us at all. However, in no sense do we think of her as handicapped.
>
> (Ablon, 1990: 884)

And, in another interview, one respondent says:

> He gets on the subway with a special ticket. It's for senior citizens, kids under 10, and the handicapped.
> [Does it bother him if he gets on the subway with his friends and they pull out a white ticket and he has a red ticket?]
> No. But he refused to get in the handicapped gym class because he said 'I'm not handicapped.'
> [Who was in the class?]
> Somebody who has arthritis, and there are people with wheelchairs. He said, 'I'm not getting in the handicapped gym class. I'm not handicapped.'

[Then why would he use the red ticket?]
It's cheaper and it doesn't seem to bother him.
[Would it bother you to use the term handicapped for him?]
No. The fact is he is handicapped in certain situations where he's just got limitations, and that's all there is to it. He can't do certain things.

(Ablon, 1990: 884)

It is only social scientists who assume that it is meaningful to place people in fixed categories. In practice, labels tend to be used strategically to achieve particular contextually bounded outcomes. The politics of language use is complex and reflects the reality that categorisations shift according to the pragmatic needs of the person speaking.

The next section of this chapter moves from a discussion of language *use* to an analysis of discursive *structures*. It looks at the linguistic construction of two categories of 'impairment' – 'madness' and 'stupidity' – in order to interrogate the historical production of certain kinds of differences.

Structuring 'madness'

We tend to think of 'madness' and 'sanity' as being two quite clear-cut and distinct states. We also tend to treat madness as a state of irrationality suffered by certain people who have particular constitutions or have had painful emotional experiences. In the modern era, Western societies have designed a number of ways of classifying and treating 'the mad'. Institutions and professions have developed to care for and cure the mad, and accounts of the 'history of madness' offer a story or picture of growing humanity in the treatment of such people.

However what if, as Parker *et al.* (1995) ask,

the very act of dividing reason from unreason were a product of culture? ... We need some understanding of the cultural production of the rational as a 'good thing' and the irrational as something which needs not only to be excluded but also to be rigorously policed.

(Parker *et al.*, 1995: 12)

Foucault, in his groundbreaking work *Madness and Civilisation*

(1965), questioned the idea that madness can be located simply in individuals. Rather, it is a product of the technologies and knowledge involved in categorisation. Foucault showed how, with the advent of the Enlightenment, the voice of 'unreason' was silenced and excluded. In order to silence such voices, 'the mad' were excluded from the public arena, and confined to institutions.

> The post-enlightenment authorities instigated the 'great confinement', taking place in France by the middle of the seventeenth century and in England in the houses of correction of the sixteenth century. The institutions of the great confinement served many purposes; to instil religious and moral virtue, to absorb the labour of the unemployed, and finally by the nineteenth century, as the temple of medical science wherein the new profession of psychiatry developed its administrative methods, psychological theories and taxonomic schemes.
>
> (Sampson, 1994: 56)

The repressive power that segregated the mad was thus embodied within the architecture of the asylum. From the nineteenth century, 'hospitals became predicated on the moral and physical architecture of Jeremy Bentham's Panopticon – literally spaces where patients could be seen, observed and controlled' (Sampson, 1994: 57). As psychiatry and psychology developed categories of madness, so groups of people were 'identified' and labelled as belonging to these categories[1]. In other words, the development of categories of madness followed from the development of architectural spaces and the new uses which were made of them. Once the categories and administrative procedures existed, a new and expanding population of 'mad' people were discovered to fill these spaces. The voices of the mad were silenced. One of Foucault's concerns was to resist 'disciplinary' discourses and give space for local knowledge and the repressed voice of unreason.

Examination of the *Diagnostic and Statistical Manual* (DSM) of the American Association of Psychiatrists provides a very clear example of the way in which madness is historically and culturally contingent. New disorders are constantly being 'discovered' (in recent years, post-traumatic stress disorder and attention deficit disorder) and old disorders can be withdrawn from the category of the pathological. In 1973, the American Psychiatric Association's Board of Trustees voted to take 'Ego-dystonic homosexuality' off its list of mental illnesses, and the American Psychological Association followed suit two years later (Parker *et al.*, 1995). Whilst the American Psychiatric Association would defend the change on the grounds of growing scientific understanding, is was also influenced by the campaigning of gay organisations. It is also true that new conditions are frequently accepted into official classifications as a result of campaigning for recognition. Whilst emotional distress (or mental illness) clearly exists, the way in which it is identified and classified may say more about the processes of categorisation than the 'underlying reality'.

By showing that madness is not simply 'discovered', but is rather constituted in large part by the psychiatric profession, which has the power to police populations and apply labels, Foucault drew attention to the work of professional bodies in constituting a range of pathologies. Such professionals need technological, administrative and architectural resources to perform their tasks of categorising and treating people. Knowledge about madness cannot be separated from the power to intervene in observing, investigating and treating 'mad' people.

It is important to note the way in which the categories of madness interact with other social categorisations based, for example on gender and 'race'. For example, black people and women are more likely to be hospitalised for schizophrenia (Fernando, 1991). Goldberg and Huxley have noted that 'with few exceptions, most studies show greater rates for common mental disorders in those of lower [sic] social class' (1992: 19). Far from engaging in value-neutral procedures for measurement and treatment, psychiatry reflects social and cultural prejudices.

Another example of a category of 'disability' which is discursively constituted, is the category of stupidity.

Constituting stupidity

What do the terms 'imbecile', 'cretin', 'moron' and 'feeble-minded' have in common? The first answer might be that they are all used as terms of abuse. Another answer is that they are all official terms, enshrined in UK legislation, to refer to people who are deemed to fall below a standard category of general 'educability' (Solity, 1992). Nowadays, those pupils who are seen as having additional requirements that are not being met by mainstream education are identified as having 'special educational needs'. The identification, classification and treatment of 'learning disabilities', as with mental illness, is similarly not a value-free process. The way in which intellectual impairments are identified changes constantly (Tomlinson, 1981; Swann, 1986; Bowman, 1986). Whilst most societies have in the past had some members who were considered a bit slow, and who may have grown up to be the 'village idiots' (see Groce, 1992), it was not until the introduction of universal education that the category of 'ineducable' was medically defined and deployed as the basis for segregation. In 1924, the Wood Committee on mental deficiency in the UK recommended that the 'defective, dull and backward' should be envisaged as a single group presenting a single educational and administrative problem. This group was subsequently termed educationally subnormal (ESN) (Tomlinson, 1981: 43).

The criteria for identifying educational subnormality were the outcome of performance in an intelligence test. Yet the whole process of intelligence testing can be seen as constructed. Pupils were tested and their scores placed upon a linear scale. Those pupils falling in the bottom percentiles, with an IQ score of below 70, were defined as being educationally subnormal. Cyril Burt, the educational psychologist who developed this cut-off point did so by working out the numbers of pupils who could be accommodated within special education. As such, the number of pupils in the subnormal category says more about the arbitrary cut-off point for those receiving educational provision than about any natural dividing line between groups of pupils. Despite Burt being personally discredited for using fraudulent data and for intelligence testing generally having social and cultural biases (Rose et al., 1984), intelligence tests remain a central tool in the assessment of educability. The 1981 Education Act defined learning difficulties as having a 'significantly greater difficulty in learning than the majority of children' (Croll et al., 1984: 146). It suggested that one in five pupils will have some form of special educational need. This figure reproduces the purely pragmatic figure employed by Burt for determining provision.

As in the case of mental illness, the people identified as having learning difficulties are not distributed evenly through the population. This is particularly the case for those identified as having moderate learning difficulties (in which, generally, no organic cause has been identified). Working-class boys are much more likely to be seen as having learning difficulties than middle-class girls and boys (Collier, 1987). Black boys are more likely to be classified as having an emotional-behavioural difficulty than black girls or white pupils (Tomlinson, 1982).

What we learn from the examples of madness and learning difficulties is the importance of interrogating the procedures by which labels are developed and applied to people, and the ways in which certain differences are constituted as salient in particular historical and social settings. Once we have recognised that labels cannot be taken for granted as referring to essential differences, then it is possible to contest some of the diagnostic claims made by some professionals.

Some people see the term 'learning difficulties' as qualitatively different from previous terminological changes, since it is the term chosen by organised groups, such as People First. It is a proud self-definition rather than a category imposed from outside. We can see a similar process in the gay liberation movement, which has held on to the term 'gay' as a respectful and positive term.

The next section of this chapter therefore looks at some of the ways disabled people have attempted to take control over the language of disability. Self-representation lies at the heart of the disabled people's movement. Disabled people have deployed two main strategies in the struggle to resist offensive disablist terminology. These can be described as 'positive naming' and 'defiant self-naming'.

Positive naming

Positive naming deploys terms which either have positive connotations or which confine the negative aspects of terms to a specific impairment – rather than allowing it to engulf the disabled persons whole identity. A good example of the positive naming strategy can be found in the UK Spastics Society decision to change its name to Scope. The reason for this change is because the term 'spastic', originally purely a medical description of the condition cerebral palsy, had become contaminated with highly offensive connotations. 'Spastic' had become so widespread a term of abuse, that there was no way of 'rescuing it' as an acceptable description of people with cerebral palsy. Scope gives the following account of its name change: 'We changed because our name was offensive and hurtful to the people we work with. We have become Scope because the name represents what we work to achieve – scope for people to live the life they choose' (Scope 1995). Scope offers a list of 'positive' and 'negative' words. For example, Scope suggest that 'people with disabilities' and 'disabled people' are positive, whilst 'the disabled' and 'cripples' should be avoided. Another example of an important contribution to the positive language debate is made by Shearer (1996). She writes, 'there is no such thing as a neutral image of a person who has a mental handicap. Unless it is deliberately made positive, people will see it as confirming their negative preconceptions – whether that is intended or not' (Shearer, 1996: 205).

The point of the positive language debate is that it suggests changes in terminology which alter perceptions of disabled people by focusing on capacities rather than limitations, and differences rather than deviance. The medical sociologist and disability activist Irving K. Zola supports such strategies because they treat disabilities as verbs rather than nouns. Zola argues that people have multiple roles and that they should not be 'reduced' to their disability. He suggests that in language, 'the disability and the person remain separate' (Zola, 1988: 379). The 'positive' naming approach sits well with the pluralistic culture of the USA. People with impairments are sometimes referred to as being 'differently abled'.

There have been a number of criticisms of 'positive' naming. Terms which refer to disabled people as a 'challenge', either to others (e.g. the badly behaved child who is a 'challenge to the services') or to themselves (e.g. the short person who is 'vertically challenged'), are derided as being euphemistic and ridiculous. They deny real differences. Why should a disabled person be 'a person with a disability', when a woman is not 'a person with an X-chromosome', an old person is not 'a person who has lived a long time', or an intelligent person is not 'a person with high levels of intelligence'? All these examples indicate an attempt to appeal to the authentic and core person, underlying what are presumed to be 'superficial' aspects associated with physical or intellectual appearance or functioning. An attempt is made to put the 'person first', because it is assumed that the impairment is so negative that it eclipses personhood. A linguistic alteration is seen as overcoming this difficulty.

Defiant self-naming

Perhaps the ultimate back-handed 'compliment' is to say to a disabled person, 'I don't think of you as disabled.' It presumes that to think of someone as disabled is to think badly of them. The concern among the disabled people's movement is to achieve acceptance as a disabled person. Disabled people should not be required to disguise or 'overcome' their impairment or any difficulties associated with it. Such pride does not necessarily involve saying 'I'm glad I had polio [or], Don't you wish you were blind' (see Zola, 1985). Rather, pride is about achieving acceptance and respect for people, whatever their 'dis/ability' status.

One way for achieving recognition of difference is to 'come out', in a strategy analogous to that taken by many lesbian and gay people. This may involve reappropriating previously offensive terminology as ironic self-description. In much the same way as the gay community has reappropriated the term 'queer' to refer to a specific strand of gay culture, disabled people might call themselves 'crips'. Such language rejects 'positive' euphemism. It also contains an important element of 'in-your-face' confrontation with non-disabled people. As Mairs writes,

> People – crippled or not – wince at the word cripple, as they do not at handicapped or disabled. Perhaps I want them to wince. I want them to see me as a tough customer, one to whom the fates/gods/viruses have not been kind, but who can face the brutal truth of her existence squarely. As a cripple, I swagger.
>
> (Mairs, 1986: 9)

Open display of difference is thus a political act which challenges the 'normals' who may well feel uncomfortable with such language. Reclaiming terminology has value in being resistant to non-disabled appropriation, since it would not be acceptable for a non-disabled person to use the language of 'crips' unless they were in a position of great trust and involvement with disabled people. All too often the reason new terms take on offensive connotations is because they are used in the same way as previous terms. Self-naming is protected from colonisation by non-disabled people. The concern to achieve acceptance of differences is considered by Zola in his appraisal of marathon running. He argues that it is the only sport where people with a disability can fully participate on their own terms:

> It is not accidental that marathon running is the only sport where people with disabilities ... have been integrated into the mainstream, not by denying their disabilities or 'overcoming them', but making them the very basis on which they compete.
>
> (Zola, 1985: 6)

When disabled people succeed in representing themselves, on their own terms, their political gains don't get incorporated back into a disablist status quo. This is because self-representation does not just alter the form which images of disability take. It also alters the relationship which non-disabled and disabled people have to the symbolic universe.

Despite the positive values associated with fostering pride and celebrating difference, Shakespeare identifies certain risks:

> While the disability movement seeks inclusion and integration, it also celebrates difference. The margins are a good place to speak from, and there is a cost to coming into the mainstream. But celebrating and identifying in difference can be a risk – for example, recuperating the term 'cripple': 'The dangerous intimacy between subjectification and subjection needs careful calibration' (Riley, 1988, p.17).
>
> (Shakespeare *et al.*, 1996: 106)

Whilst positive terminology offers temporary comforts, celebrating difference and reclaiming previously offensive terminology is a strategy of struggle which places the problem of language in a central position.

In the next part of the chapter, I will outline some further dangers inherent in the use of positive terminology, which seems to defer rather than resolve the problem of disablist language.

Unconscious investments

Having identified two strategies – adopting positive terminology and asserting difference – in this section I discuss some of the unconscious meanings and effects of these strategies.

Euphemism

'Updating' language is one of the key ways in which disability professionals attempt to distinguish themselves from their predecessors. Politically correct terminology establishes the credentials of the user as someone who has achieved enlightenment. By denigrating previous ways of speaking, people can take a superior stance that prevents them from looking critically at themselves and the complex ways in which language functions. Sinason, however, offers an analysis which can help us to think about this 'linguistic inflation'. She writes:

> Each worker introducing a new term hopes that the new word brings new hope and a new period of historical change. Each time the new word is coined, it is coined honourably. ... Each such chapter praises itself for its hopeful new term. It is therefore doing a grave disservice to past pioneers to point contemptuously to their chosen term.
>
> (Sinason, 1992: 40)

Thus, when Sinason joined Symington's 'subnormality workshop', she and a colleague, Jon Stokes, changed the name to the 'mental handicap workshop'. They felt disdain towards those using the word 'subnormal'. However, a few years later, 'learning disability' became the new and politically approved term. Suddenly, those using 'handicap' were seen as being oppressive. It was at this point that Sinason came to realise that changes in terminology can reflect a process of euphemism rather than a change in underlying assumptions.

Euphemisms are needed when something uncomfortable and difficult cannot be faced and so needs to be disguised. Thus, when someone working as a professional with disabled people refers to their 'client', the term may appear to accord respect, yet in practice it may function to disguise the lack of choice regarding the services being offered. Davis writes that it is

> interesting and instructive to reflect on why it is that these people have decided to call us their 'clients' ... they may say that 'client' is a nice easy word, which avoids the anonymity of 'person' or 'disabled person'. ... Or that 'client' gives a disabled person some dignity, some status. That more recent one is particularly pleasing, as it conveys the idea of equality wrapped up in more recent connotations which assign consumer status to both patron and client. A very neat bit of professional sleight of speech, suggesting equivalence in choice and control, even though they and we know that the reality is very different ... they need to contain their dominance and our dependence within a coherent philosophical framework designed to encapsulate, reinforce and sustain the interests of the industry. Such a framework needs to be flexible enough to move with the times,

keep abreast of public sympathy, but ensure that their control over our lives remains essentially untouched. Thus, it has come to be that the disability 'professionals' and us, their 'clients', live within the carefully crafted, mechanical embrace of 'care'.

(Davis, 1994: 198–9)

A young woman with Down's syndrome offered a mischievous parody of professional terminology in her announcement to Sinason at the start of her therapy session: 'I've got four handicaps. I've got Down's syndrome, special needs, learning disability and a mental handicap' (Sinason, 1998).

Davis and the young woman with 'four handicaps' both demonstrate that the panoply of labels professionals use function in a way which is alienating to the recipients. The labels serve to avoid acknowledgement of power differences. Politically correct language can be seen as just another device with which to reinforce hierarchy between professional groups. Some professionals may use the most up-to-date language in order to compete with other professionals and appear 'more politically correct than thou' (Marks, 1996b). The arrogance and contempt which proponents of politically correct language sometimes appear to have for their predecessors, and the language they employ boomerangs back to them when a new even more up-to-date person comes along.

As Sinason puts it, 'euphemisms, linguistically are brought in to replace the verbal bedlinen when a particular word feels too raw, too near a disturbing experience' (1992: 40). Sinason argues that instead of acknowledging real differences and difficulties faced by people with learning difficulties, there is an attempt to deny such differences. At an unconscious level, she is suggesting that the constant changing of terms expresses a desire to make the impairment go away. In this way, 'positive terminology' can serve as denial rather than acceptance of disabled people. Euphemistic terminology, such as 'differently abled' seems to deny any impairment or difficulty. As Wolfensberger puts it:

Terms virtually drip with surplus meaning when they become out-and-out code words, far removed from the face validity of the term itself. ... For instance, who ever would have thought that the term 'self-advocate' would come to mean largely a mentally retarded person, as in the picture caption, 'Three self-advocates having lunch,' which referred to three mentally retarded persons?

(Wolfensberger, 1994: 285)

As such, positive terminology relies on the somewhat naive assumption that language change on its own can bring about social change. As Sinason says, 'a true understanding that we are all equal souls and all handicapped in different ways gets transmuted into a manic desire to erase difference' (Sinason, 1992: 43). Whilst (unconscious) hostile and aggressive feelings are held towards those with the 'learning difficulties', new terms designed to avoid the offensive associations of previous terms will become rapidly contaminated. Again, Sinason offers a powerful description of this process when she points out that 'no human group has been forced to change its name so frequently. The sick and the poor are always with us, in physical presence and in verbal terms, but not the handicapped' (1992: 40).

Summary

Language does not refer unproblematically to an external world. We cannot know reality 'objectively', through direct perception, in the way in which empiricist epistemologists have argued. Empiricism suggests that the only thing we can really trust is the evidence of our senses. However, this fails to acknowledge the impossibility of unmediated perception. Our perceptions of the world are constituted out of the discursive resources available to us. Our 'intuitions' about needs, rights, beauty, humanity, desire and differences are socially constituted. As Turner summarises, 'what we know about "the world" is simply the outcome of arbitrary conventions we adopt to describe the world' (1995:11). It is therefore a central concern of Disability Studies to demystify the conventions operating in the organisation of knowledge about 'impairment' and 'disability'.

Language is productive, it constitutes and reproduces reality, but it also seems to be the case that attempts to change terminology will not break the negative chain of disabling associations. Language both produces and disguises meanings. As such, language is both a cause and a symptom of a disabling society.

If we suggest that changing terminology is not enough, are we suggesting that language is not important in the politics of disability?

Is there a way of attending to the constitutive nature of language without taking an idealistic position and constantly updating euphemistic categories that seem to serve merely to repress hostile and derogatory ways of representing disability? Whilst the 'turn to language' has emphasised that words are important, they must be understood within a social context of segregation, exclusion and denigrating practices.

Investments in images

Introduction

Our sense of citizenship and community is defined by boundaries which demarcate zones of inclusion and exclusion. The question of what constitutes social membership has become one of the key issues in citizenship debates (Sibley, 1996). This chapter examines the way in which these boundaries are defined and reinforced by images within popular culture. The media uses images of impairment in order to represent some of our deepest fears concerning 'normality' and 'belonging'.

Perhaps the most striking feature of contemporary images of disabled people is that they are frequently isolated and disengaged from the community. Norden's (1994) encyclopaedic book *Cinemas of Isolation* lists 600 films which have disability as a central concern. Often, disability forms an 'absent presence' within film and TV. That is, assumptions about impairments are often latent in the film and not consciously registered by the spectator as being *about* disability. Walmsley (1997) for example, argues that the threatening super-natural characters in the *X-Files* serve to constitute 'abnormal' outsiders who 'stand for' disabled people. Images of impairment function as metaphors for particular states and experiences. Norden identifies some of the key ways in which film-makers isolate disabled characters, including 'framing, editing, sound, lighting, set design elements (eg. fences, windows, staircase banisters) – [which serve] to suggest a physical or symbolic separation of disabled characters from the rest of society' (1995: 6).

This chapter explores some of the ways in which disability is constituted through the symbolic isolation of certain individuals. The approach taken, as in the previous chapter, is textual. That is, an attempt is made to *read* visual representations rather than to treat the objects of perception as prediscursive and essential. The focus of analysis is on how visual images serve to constitute particular emotional, intellectual, functional, aesthetic and spiritual qualities. It identifies the (latent) disabling 'stories' contained within images.

Cultural images of disability have been explored widely by Longmore (1987), Gartner and Joe (1987), Klobas (1988), Evans (1992), Morris (1991), Barnes (1992), Cumberbatch and Negrine (1992), Darke (1994), Norden (1994), Hevey (1992) and Garland Thompson (1996, 1997), to name but a few of the most notable works. The first part of this chapter will offer a brief introductory review of some of this work. It begins by noting the absence and presence of images of disability. It then discusses Western notions of beauty and 'normal' bodily and intellectual functioning. It looks at how visual images serve to constitute authority, dependency, savagery and innocence. The second part of the chapter connects the insights of disability scholars to psychoanalytic theorising about the management of emotional difficulties and differences. Specifically, it explores two particular socially constituted 'states' of 'stupidity' and 'monstrosity', and psychic fears and fantasies associated with these states.

Aesthetics

Dutton (1995), in his analysis of the shifts in Western consciousness of the body, argues that the overwhelming preoccupation in classical Greek society, during the Italian Renaissance and also in modern popular culture has been with the search for human perfection. The ancient Greeks first formulated the question 'in what does perfection consist and further, what kind of perfection can a human being – as a human being – reach?' (Dutton, 1995: 12). Plato suggested that ideal forms provide templates for aesthetic beauty. The everyday world of the senses is surpassed by a timeless world of forms. The classical body is constituted as 'transcendent and monumental, closed, static, self-contained, symmetrical and sleek; it is identified with the 'high' or official culture of the Renaissance, and later, with rationalism, individualism, and normalising aspirations of the bourgeoisie' (Russo, 1995: 8).

Following Platonic ideals, Western art has sought to represent the perfect human body. This has taken the form of concentration – particularly in images of the male form – on 'external activity, on outward visibility, on physical striving and action' (Dutton, 1995: 366).

Regulating and excluding bodies

Platonic notions of beauty have, in the nineteenth and twentieth centuries, become elided with social Darwinian and utilitarian notions of 'fitness' (see Williamson, 1997) to produce stringent calls to exercise control over our bodies. Cosmetic surgery, removal of bodily hair (usually for women), the use of personal trainers (for those who can afford them) to develop programmes tailored to motivate particular individuals, diet plans and a range of health and beauty treatments all call upon the modern subject to correct 'flaws' in their appearance and engage in rigorous self-discipline. In contemporary atomised society, the body is for many people one of the few remaining and direct areas of control and self-expression. Shilling writes, 'If one feels unable to exert control over an increasingly complex society, at least one can have some effect on the size, shape and appearance of one's body' (1993: 7). The body is thus used increasingly as a marker of distinction and 'an entity which is in the process of becoming; a project which should be worked at and accomplished as part of an individual's self-identity' (Shilling, 1993: 5).

Shaban (1996) sees such policing practices, and the subsequent denigration of those bodies which do not conform to ideals, as expressing a form of 'body fascism'. Disabled characters (not just in films but also in print journalism, TV and advertising) are often portrayed as 'overcoming' their impairment. Portraying the striving of such courageous people (e.g. Christie Brown in the movie *My Left Foot*), who are often referred to in the disability literature as the 'Supercrips' (Shaban, 1996), functions to blame disabled people for their limitations (Morris, 1991). This is because the implicit message is that if these courageous people could triumph over their impairments, then those who fail to achieve great things have less courage and are perhaps responsible for their pitiful lives. Sometimes even the ability to regain functioning is attributed to heroic effort on the part of the individual concerned and his or her non-disabled companions or doctors. Perhaps there is a difficulty in acknowledging that some impairments cannot be removed through sheer force of will and determination. Disabled people thus function as an uncomfortable reminder that we may not be in total control of our destiny, and that our bodies and minds are vulnerable to damage. As Zola puts it,

> With society raging against such 'killer' diseases ... should it be a surprise that some of the anger at the diseases spills over onto the bearers of diseases? To some, those with physical and mental disabilities become objects, the permanent reminders of a lost or losing struggle, the symbols of a past and continuing failure. America likes winners. It forgets, denies, rejects and neglects losers.
>
> (Zola, 1988: 373)

The work of constructing the modern body relies on a series of exclusions, since we can only know what is a 'fit' and 'attractive' body if we have a concept of an 'unfit' and 'unattractive' body. As Haraway states, 'what counts as human and as non-human is not given by definition, but only by relation, by engagement in situated, worldly encounters, where boundaries take shape and categories sediment' (Haraway, 1994: 64). Goffman shows how important visual markers are in securing the exclusion of particular individuals. He begins his book *Stigma* by referring to the way in which the ancient Greeks concretely marked a socially devalued trait.

> The Greeks, who were apparently strong on visual aids, originated the term stigma to refer to bodily signs designed to expose something unusual and bad about the moral status of the signifier. The signs were cut or burnt into the body and advertised that the bearer was a slave, a criminal, or a traitor – a blemished person, ritually polluted.
>
> (Goffman, 1963: 11)

This external demonstration of 'internal blemish' was an important theme in the work of nineteenth-century evolutionary psychologists and phrenologists such as Cesare Lombroso, who became engaged in a project of classifying abnormality by identifying 'correlations' between external appearance and 'criminality' (Young, 1970).

Displaying bodies

Such pseudo-scientific concerns were reflected in nineteenth-century popular culture, such as 'freak shows':

As a cultural representation in the late Nineteenth Century, the freak belongs to the increasingly codified world of the spectacle. ... More than merely an image or collection of images, the spectacle is a way of looking, a world vision which has become objectified.

(Russo, 1995: 79)

Bogdan argues that 'freak' is not a quality that belongs to the person on display. Rather, it is something that we have created: 'a perspective, a set of practices – a social construction' (1988: xi). The context is set by developing racialised discourses which constitute and regulate differences, and construct a certain 'gaze' (as discussed in Chapter 3), which produces the abnormal and exotic subject. However, Bogdan also goes on to identify a whole industry of fakery, including photographing 'dwarfs' in oversize chairs and 'giants' in scaled-down chairs, fat people stuffed with padding, the doctoring of negatives and the use of a range of 'authentifications' from doctors, scientists and public officials. There is an obsessive fascination with 'Otherness', to the extent that it must be demonstrated – even by exaggeration.

Whilst the formal display of 'freaks' for entertainment in the form of the freak show is no longer with us, visual markers continue to be used in popular culture in the classification of abnormality. Unofficial freak shows take the form of 'human interest' journalism, confessional TV and medical documentaries. Even in terms of issues of political leadership, visual images play an important part in qualifying individuals for fitness to hold office.

Constituting authority and 'ability'

Models of authority play an important role in reproducing the status quo. The question asked by an 11-year-old girl towards the end of Margaret Thatcher's thirteen-year rule as British prime minister – 'can a man be Prime Minister?' – is highly instructive. Our sense of how things are is so easy to naturalise into how things should or will always be. We might ask a similar question about disabled people. Can disabled people reach the highest public office? If we examine images of leaders, it becomes clear that despite the ending of European divine monarchy, the body continues to be held up as a symbol of society (Douglas, 1991 [1966]). If a person is perceived to have a damaged or unreliable body, then they are not seen as a strong leader. When Jimmy Carter collapsed during a run and Neil Kinnock slipped during an election campaign these accidents were public relations setbacks. When leaders have had some substantial physical impairment, elaborate efforts are made to prevent it from becoming apparent to the population.

Thus, even in the sphere of political authority it is clear that again and again it has been found necessary to disguise impairment for fear that the suggestion of disability, however irrelevant to the work in hand, might undermine the authority of the politician. Gallagher (1985) shows how President Roosevelt developed a carefully orchestrated strategy to disguise the extent of his paralysis. Roosevelt was a paraplegic, as a result of childhood polio. He needed to present himself as a person who could (literally) stand on his own two feet. Roosevelt could only 'walk' with the aid of leg braces, which could be locked in a standing position. When walking he would hold his arm at a rigid ninety degree angle, often supported by his son on one arm and using a stick on the other. Gallagher describes this system of walking as 'treacherous, slow and awkward'. Roosevelt employed other strategies, such as arriving first in a meeting so he could be seated before others arrived. He only used a wheelchair in private. He was never lifted in public, and the secret service would intervene if any photographers attempted to take photos which showed the extent of his paralysis. (There are over thirty-five thousand still photographs of FDR at the Presidential Library but only two of him seated in his wheelchair: Gallagher, 1985.) Further, there are no newsreel films showing him being carried or pushed. In fact, many of them present him as a man of action.

> Wherever he went, the Secret Service went first. ... upon occasion the Secret Service would actually raise the entire level of a street to the level of the building entrance by means of temporary but extensive wooden trestles and scaffolding.
>
> (Gallagher, 1985: 97)

Roosevelt's biographers perpetuated the myth that his illness was merely an 'episode' from which he recovered. His 'triumph' over polio was seen as 'paralleling the USA's recovery and triumph from the Depression'. The impression is given that

Roosevelt gets polio, struggles through his rehabilitation and then overcomes his adversity. End of chapter. The handicap is not mentioned again. It is viewed only as one of the stages through which FDR passes in preparation for the presidency.

(Gallagher, 1985: 210)

Having identified such 'Herculean' efforts to 'embody normalcy' (Davis, 1995: 98), it is also important to explore the construction of abnormality.

Performing disability

Disabled people are, by virtue of their impairments, accorded stereotyped or even iconic (see Darke, 1997) status. It is very rare for an impairment to be presented as an incidental characteristic, which has no more significance to character and storyline than hair or eye colour. The portrayal of impairment on TV does not reflect the statistical incidence of impairment within wider society. This is particularly true in soap operas and dramas where there tend to be very few people with serious impairments (Longmore, 1987). This is, to be fair, also true for a wide range of other groups. Old women tend not to be portrayed as sexually active in movies and news-readers are never very fat – indeed, if they are women, they tend to be quite slim and attractive. TV generally does not reflect a cross-section of the population. It both reflects and reinforces racialised, gendered and cultural prejudices.

However, whilst in some genres disabled people are absent, in other media disability forms a central, although often latent, element in the story. A great number of movies, documentaries and 'human interest' stories are concerned with disability. What is significant is that these stories tend to be framed by non-disabled people as experts, relatives or even actors playing disabled people. In the ten-year period between 1981 and 1991, seven Oscars were won by non-disabled actors playing disabled people (Gullo, 1991). Examples of winners include Dustin Hoffman in *Rain Man*, Al Pacino in *Scent of a Woman*, Tom Hanks in *Forrest Gump* and Daniel Day Lewis in *My Left Foot*. The director Alex Cox, in a recent radio documentary asked a number of directors why they continue to use non-disabled people to play disabled characters? Some responded that acting is all about pretending. Make-up is used to age charac-ters, and depressed, fit and ugly actors can play happy, unfit and beautiful characters, so why shouldn't non-disabled people play disabled people? However this apparently reasonable explanation would not be acceptable if used to justify white people 'blacking up'. Many directors responded to Cox's question by saying that there is a shortage of disabled actors. Yet Equity has a list of 500 disabled actors. There are also a number of innovative disabled people's acting companies such as Graeae and Strathcona in the UK, and similar companies in the USA. The lack of experience among disadvantaged groups has long been used as a justification of restricting access to prized jobs.

Perhaps the real reason for not employing disabled people is that it is reassuring for the viewer to know that 'it's only pretend'. This point perhaps gets to the heart of the problem since it indicates that there is a positive taboo on using disabled people to play disabled parts. Disabled characters function as objects available to receive the projections of non-disabled viewers, who can observe them from a safe distance, reassured in that knowledge that 'Al Pacino isn't really blind' and 'Leonardo Di Caprio (in *What's Eating Gilbert Grape*) isn't autistic'. As such, portrayals of disability are cathartic, offering a way for non-disabled people to express their fears and fantasies of lack, dependency and loss at one remove. If the actor was disabled, then their continued existence after the movie would act as a continued reminder of these feared states.

An impossible life: the noble savage

Disabled people, like women and racialised minorities, are frequently portrayed as being 'closer to nature'. The film *The Elephant Man*, directed by David Lynch, offers an interesting example of such a construction. The film portrays the life story of John Merrick, who was born in 1862, and who began to develop a swelling (inside his lower lip) at the age of 21 months. Throughout his childhood a number of physical protrusions developed so that by early adulthood his whole body was severely deformed. Darke's (1994) review of Lynch's movie of Merrick's life identifies a number of devices to convey what he describes as a surreal sense of John Merrick being the product of 'bestial' and 'unnatural' intercourse. In the opening scene of the film, Merrick's mother is knocked down by an elephant whilst she is in the early stages of pregnancy. This event, which did occur in real life, was seen by Merrick's mother (and in the absence of a medical diagnosis explaining his condition) as being the cause of her son's deformities. The 'folkloric belief in maternal imprinting – that is [that] a psychological fright or trauma can be transmitted into a physical effect on the child in the womb' was seen, at the time, as being as good as any other explanation (Ford, 1997: 3). Darke argues that by choosing to use the elephant image in the film's opening scene, Lynch presents a sense of impending abnormality and supports the metaphysical notion of 'maternal imprinting' as an explanation for Merrick's condition. Yet whilst on the one hand Lynch reinforces such superstition, he also takes an uncritical position of support for medicine, which is presented as relatively humane.

The film portrays a series of moves in Merrick's life, from abuse at the hands of his cruel family and the workhouse, via degeneration and exploitation in the hands of lower-class exploitative show people, to sanctuary in the hands of middle- and upper-class rescuers, who nevertheless have their own voyeuristic and ambitious motivations. In all these stages of his life, Merrick is portrayed as a victim, who nevertheless survives such external horrors by functioning on a higher spiritual plane, appreciating the simple pleasures in life and somehow operating beyond the selfish interests of those around him. At the end of the film Merrick is portrayed as ending his tragic life by lying down – a 'normal' position which had not been possible for Merrick because the weight of his head made breathing impossible. Darke (1994) argues that there is no evidence that John Merrick made this Christ-like sacrifice to end his life. The cinematic decision by Lynch to present Merrick as deliberately lying down reinforces the sense of tragedy about his 'unbearable' existence. One is left with the sense that (as with Don McLean's song, *Vincent*) 'this world was never meant for one as beautiful' (in the spiritual sense of the word) as him.

The killing off of disabled characters reflects an ambivalence towards disabled people's existence. One can identify similar ambivalence in the portrayal of male characters with learning 'disabilities'. They are often seen as being more intuitive, 'childlike', spontaneous and innocent and also – the other side of the same coin – uncivilised, unpredictable and dangerous. In films such as *Of Mice and Men*, *What's Eating Gilbert Grape*, *Rain Man*, *Forrest Gump* and *Sling Blade*, the learning disabled characters are concerned and humane, yet also lack understanding and behave in ways that threaten both themselves and others. It is significant that all these characters are men who represent a version of masculine desire without access to sexual rewards. There is often a pretty woman who is admired or even idealised by the disabled character who is not available to him. Whilst these learning disabled characters are portrayed with great sympathy, they are also seen as being capable of causing great damage. As a consequence, there is usually no way in which they can be integrated into 'normal' society. Learning disabled characters rarely develop, either emotionally or in terms of their social position, through the course of the film. Often, the film ends locating them at the same place that they began. In *Rain Man* and *Sling Blade*, the learning disabled character returns to the institution he lived in at the beginning of the film. The message here is that despite dreams of inclusion, there is only one place for them.

Idealising disabled characters for their 'childlike goodness' thus occurs in tandem with denigrating them. Klein (1952) shows that idealisation is a psychic mechanism that functions as a defence against destructive instincts. The aggressive desire to remove the recipient of hostile projections (by killing them or sending them to an institution) is split off and disavowed. The 'object' is endowed with earthly dangers (such as sexual desire and aggression) and spiritual virtues (childlike innocence and goodness) which are then used as a receptacle for the non-disabled viewers' projections.

The portrayal of disabled people as 'closer to nature' is also found in the film and play *Children of a Lesser God*. Sandhal (1991) outlines its implicit disablist assumptions. The story is about a romantic relationship between Sarah, who is deaf and works as a caretaker in the school for the deaf (in which she was once a student), and James, a new member of staff at the school. The couple engage in a 'battle of wills', in which Sarah refuses to speak and insists on signing. The perspective which the play adopts is that of James, who is concerned to investigate Sarah's past by visiting her mother and reading her files. The implication is that only psychological trauma can explain Sarah's refusal to learn to speak, rather than any kind of political resistance to hearing culture. James' love and understanding for Sarah enable her to adjust to her past. Ultimately, he represents a civilising influence on Sarah. She learns to speak and they marry.

As a version of Rousseau's 'noble savage' and Said's 'exotic oriental', Sandhal shows that Sarah supports a myth of the feminine as 'Other' to the rational Western civilised man. Sarah's silence gives her a sense of mystery and 'Otherness'. She has an 'uninhibited' sexuality and a 'natural' feel for musical vibrations. Such colonial images place Sarah as available to be explored and won by

James. Sarah's impairment thus becomes a metaphor for thinking about sexual relationships and psychological damage. Thus disability functions to constitute 'ability'. It is only by defining an 'Other' – someone who is fundamentally different – that non-disabled culture is able to sustain an image of itself as rational, in control, authoritative and knowing.

The exoticisation of disability also occurs in documentaries which follow a 'strange but true' format. This is particularly the case with scientific and medical documentaries which address rare 'malfunctioning' people with 'tragic' conditions, such as conjoined twins. Often the focus is on the high-technology treatments which will enable such 'curiosities' to live a 'normal' life. Such documentaries see the task a case presents as purely a technical one, involving separating flesh and organs, rather than one involving human relationships and values. The question of whether an impairment could be accepted or even valued is rarely raised. Conjoined twins represent a challenge to individuality, which is highly prized within contemporary modern society. We can make comparisons between the documentary portrayal of impairment and the portrayal of 'native peoples' within anthropology, who are presented as objects of curiosity and sometimes, also of pity.

Charity 'cripples' and other victims

Disabled people (and particularly disabled children) are often presented as tragic victims. The disabled child represents a staple of charity advertising. Dickensian images of the helpless, pure and innocent Tiny Tim character, or what Kriegel (1969) calls 'the charity cripple', evoke pity. Such sentimental characters rarely face the camera and their eyes are deferentially downcast. Apart from a recent campaign launched by Benetton (Toscani, 1998), which used images of children and young people with Down's syndrome, and an edition of *Dazed and Confused*, which contained a fashion shoot guest edited by Alexander McQueen using disabled models, disabled people are rarely used in glossy style images or commercial advertising. Two further exceptions to this are 'in-house' health service or educational magazines, where 'aids' to assist disabled people are advertised (Hevey, 1992).

Hevey (1992, 1997) offers a powerful critique of charity advertising photography. His starting point is to argue that charities function to support the grandiosity of non-disabled people, who speak 'for' disabled people and present disabled people in demeaning ways. Often realistic documentary styles are used to naturalise and give scientific credibility to the argument being made. As Evans puts it:

> documentary modes of representation ... in connoting fidelity to the Real, are damaging those they purport to represent and can be understood as the rhetorical construction of people as essential types thus securing a fixity of their status as fundamentally other, an otherness which is already long established in the name of medical science.
>
> (Evans, 1992: 45)

Evans' (1988) analysis of a charity advert (Figure 2) offers a graphic demonstration of the realist mode of presentation:

The advert features a man and a woman sitting together, locked in each other's arms. Above the picture is the text 'No sense, no feeling' and below the picture the rebuttal, 'they may not think as fast but they feel as deeply'. Evans shows how this picture presents the disabled people as aspiring to 'normal' relationships, and yet the poster functions to parody this ideal state of marital unity. She writes:

> the couple are isolated as specimens and seem to be emerging from a black background; they are photographed by a wide-angled lens which when used in close-up projects lips, noses, and hands into the viewer's space. The use of top-lighting from a small source casts deep shadows into their eyes and under their chins and emphasises the creases in their already rucked clothing. The lighting and the wide-angle lens together create the effect used typically in Gothic horror films. Furthermore the man has a pocket full of combs, implying an obsessional activity, but this paradoxically offset by both heads of hair being untidy and uncombed. Such is the handicapped character; people who are perhaps mad, certainly very peculiar, who are masquerading as normal by aspiring to the honorific portrait and the institution of marriage. Unfortunately the grimness of this ambiguous image was, in the context of the street, reinforced by its juxtaposition with colourful posters advertising an ideal world of commodity products. The text of the poster acts as a catalyst for the viewer to make an association

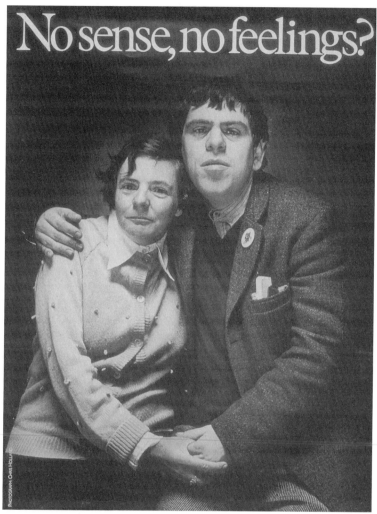

No sense, no feelings?

Figure 2   Charity advert

with the way that animal protectors refer to animals as being unable to speak, but defending them as having feelings never-theless.

(Evans, 1988: 46)

Recent adverts used by the charity in question[1] have moved away from such gritty realist presentations to offering more empowering colour images, often involving photographs taken by people with learning difficulties of other disabled people engaged in social activities with each other. Evans' analysis of the advert, and other critical deconstruction's of charity advertising (Hevey, 1992) have perhaps played a part in effecting such a policy change.

One common counter-argument to the critique of charity advertising is that the use of pitiful images of disabled people raises money for good causes, and this end justifies the means. However, Hevey has pointed out that in many of the high-profile, day-long charity events such as the Telethon,

> taking the sum of the entire voluntary donations given to the UK charitable sector, these events often raise less per day (i.e. per event) than the national daily average! Clearly, on any criterion and from any position, 'spectaculars' can't even do what they set out to do, let alone come anywhere near servicing the real needs of disabled people.
>
> (Hevey, 1992: 19)

Hevey argues that charity functions to support a society which is based on the unequal distribution of wealth, and where tax concessions offered to donors rather than redistribution of resources maintain an unequal status quo. Moreover, charities are legally bound not to engage in politics, so they are often prevented from challenging the causes of the difficulties they are organised to address. The image of the person making the appeal (the beautiful and bountiful celebrity) is as central to what charities 'do' as what is done for the recipients of donations,

Finally, charity relies on evoking feelings of pity. Lacan warns of the sense of superiority implicit in expressions of pity. 'Only saints are sufficiently detached from the deepest of the common passions to avoid the aggressive reactions to charity' (Lacan, 1977: 13). Similarly, Fenichel argues that 'pity is undoubtedly a character trait connected with an original sadism. ... This suspicion is confirmed often enough when, through analysis ... the basic mechanism appears to be an identification with the object of the original sadism' (Fenichel, 1990: 476).

Fenichel is suggesting that pity originates in a disavowal of those parts of the self which are identified in another. The pitiful disabled characters initially evoke hostile feelings because they have come to represent experiences – such as vulnerability and dependency –

which have been repressed in the spectator. These hostile feelings are quickly transformed, by a 'magical gesture', into guilt and attempts to secure forgiveness (Fenichel, 1990).

Charities tend only to exist because of socially constructed dependency in a society which fails to address the needs of disabled citizens. Further, by demeaning disabled people, charities reinforce prejudice against disabled people and thus perpetuate their exclusion. Yet having made this critique of charity, it is important not to overstate the case. Whilst accepting the unconscious sadism and narcissism behind expressions of pity, it is important to recognise that charity also involves a *reparative* intent. Just because an act may emerge as a way of resolving negative unconscious conflicts does not mean that this act does not also have valuable outcomes. The point I am making here is that we need not condemn all acts of charity as damaging to the recipient. Some charities are run by disabled people, and some have established empowering collaborations with their recipients. Since the early 1990s an increasing number of alliances have developed between organisations of disabled people and the big UK charities such as Mencap, Radar and Scope, which are increasingly adopting a rights-based approach. Indeed,

> the majority of Scope's ruling board are now disabled. Mencap has declared that people with learning disabilities will be more involved in the charity's work. Even the arch-traditional Leonard Cheshire, which runs a network of homes and services for more than 10,000 disabled people, has set up a user's group.
>
> (Benn, 1998: 4)

Further, we should not deny the possibility that individuals may be motivated by genuine acts of empathy and concern rather than pity.

Despite this caveat, the general point that acts of charity often objectify the people is an important one. Where the investments of the giver are not acknowledged it becomes all too easy to use charity as a means of resolving unconscious conflicts.

Representing evil and anger

Disability is frequently used to stand for some internal aberration or sin. Often, such badness is marked in the form of disfigurement, as in the James Bond movies. Other villains, such as Captain Hook and Richard III, plot and scheme in order to gain vengeance on a world which each sees as responsible for his wounds (Kriegel, 1969). A similar form of representation (but focusing on the bitterness rather than the evil of the 'marked' character) occurs in many post-Second World War and post-Vietnam dramas concerned with the 'returning soldier', who may represent anxiety and guilt evoked in non-disabled civilians. Such stories present disabled characters as finding it difficult to 'come to terms' with their impairments. Such characters often attempt to manipulate their non-disabled friends and family. At first, non-disabled characters feel sorry for them, and try to accommodate them. Then, they are forced to 'get tough', and give the disabled person an emotional slap around the face. The disabled person has a psychological problem of self-acceptance and the non-disabled main character helps them to achieve a better understanding of the true nature of the problem.

The soap opera, as a popular form of entertainment, is very important in both forming and reflecting attitudes. In one of the most widely watched, long-running British soap operas, *Coronation Street*, the storyline of Jim MacDonald (Summer 1998) losing the use of his legs provides an example of a particularly common stereotype. Jim becomes angry and bitter. However, with the support of his previously estranged wife Liz, and a devoted (non-disabled) occupational therapist (OT), he gradually comes to terms with his loss. Grateful for the assistance he has received and determined to get better, through sheer will-power and effort, Jim has now got back the use of his legs. However, before this happened, his wife Liz ran off with the OT and the implication is that a 'crippled' husband cannot compete with a non-disabled lover. Pity rather than desire motivated Liz' original return to Jim following his accident and her eventual dissatisfaction with him. This theme of the heroic doctor/therapist/lover/friend who, through commitment and love, is able to rescue the resentful/pitiful/dying/helpless disabled character, is a powerful and pervasive stereotype.

Assessing the significance of images of impairment

As in the context of discussions of the effects of pornography on the treatment of women, it is clear that visual representations of impairment both reflect and reinforce disablism. Given its harmful effects, should visual representations of disability always strive towards positive representations? In the previous chapter 'positive terminology' was seen as being problematic because it could take the form of euphemism which failed to address some of the underlying structural features that reproduce disability. Similarly, Darke (1997) has argued that 'negative' portrayals of disabled people may be an accurate portrayal of their social isolation and infantilisation. Darke criticises Longmore's demand for positive representations of disabled people who are portrayed occupying mainstream positions. He writes:

> Longmore is not accepting that [dependency and isolation] can be the lived reality of some disabled people. ... For me, a strand of argument that Longmore (and others) fail to take up, the discourse of what man is, is the very discourse that is used to marginalise the impaired and instigate (what Gilman (1988) calls 'self-hate') their self doubt. Such representations are not 'bad' or negative in themselves as there is nothing essentially 'wrong' (socially or culturally) in being impotent or physically dependent. ... The error of positive imagery disability writers ... is to argue that these negative portrayals should not be presented (a view Longmore leans towards). I would argue that such a philosophy only serves to marginalise those who are impotent (or the like) still further, in the hope that those who are not impotent (or physically dependent) are treated more fairly; a philosophical position that culturally reinforces the idea of normality and impairment as disability.
>
> (Darke, 1997: 37)

The main value of the critical readings by disability theorists is to offer the tools to denaturalise hegemonic discourses on impairment. Disability is not just 'out there, to be seen and understood'. Rather, it is constructed, through a range of latent visual messages. Everywhere we look, whether it is in the representations of politicians, in soap operas or movies, images of impairment are used, or more frequently misused, to define the boundaries of normality or to describe the state of 'Otherness'. Having outlined some of the overt and latent representational structures of disablement, in the next section of this chapter I explore some of the investments placed within these structures.

Psychic investments in disability

It is important to examine some of the emotional investments which function to reassure the non-disabled viewer of their 'normality'. In order to do this it is helpful to turn to psychoanalysis. What we find in analytic accounts of investments in normalcy and fears about 'stupidity' and 'monstrosity', is that those aspects of disability which generate most anxiety are precisely those areas of human experience which many people struggle with. Most of us, whatever our disability status, wonder if we are lovable and can, at times (particularly early on in life), feel excluded. Whilst such feelings tend not to be acknowledged publicly, or even consciously, having long since undergone repression, they are all too common human emotions. In the Introduction to this text, the mechanisms of repression and projection were briefly outlined. Here, it is helpful to outline some of the anxieties about identity and difference which are commonly dealt with by projection onto disabled people.

The problem of normotic tendencies

A good starting point for this discussion is to examine some of the emotional investments which get placed within categories of the 'normal'. What is it about disability that, possibly at an unconscious level, is so threatening? Why is there such a desperate desire to establish clear boundaries defining normality and abnormality?

Chrisopher Bollas offers a refreshingly critical exploration of why some individuals and cultures are so concerned to sustain the disabled/abled binary. Bollas identifies the drive towards the 'normal' as a form of illness which he terms 'normotic illness':

> A normotic person is someone who is abnormally normal. He is too stable, secure, comfortable and socially extrovert. He is fundamentally disinterested in subjective life and he is inclined to reflect on the thingness of objects, on their material reality, or on 'data' that relates to material phenomena.
>
> (Bollas, 1987: 136)

Such a person conceives their self in a similar way to a quality control department's concern with the functioning of a product. They are ultra-rational, objective, and tend to lack imagination (e.g. they speak in clichés) and empathy (they tend to steer clear of people expressing strong emotional affects). Bollas shows that the state of 'abnormal normality' is achieved by eradicating the self of subjective life. He identifies the roots of normotic illness in a failure of key attachment figures to engage in mirroring and to be responsive to a child's inner reality (discussed in Chapter 3). As Bollas puts it, 'the child is rewarded for being good, where good means ordinary, and he is ignored or threatened for being imaginative' (1987: 114). This has a deadening effect on a child's subjective world. This book is not the place to give a detailed account of the aetiology of individuals with normotic illness. However, it is important to note that whilst Bollas is primarily concerned with clinical matters, he does suggest that the normotic is a personality type emerging in contemporary culture, with its lack of empathy for certain vulnerable citizens and its drive to regulate and make normal that which is subversive, transgressive and simply different. The notion of the normotic thus seems to explain the psychic investments in the production and reproduction of normalising society.

Stupidity

Sinason identifies the etymological origins of 'stupid' as 'numbed with grief'. She argues the experience of such grief and 'the process of "going stupid" handicaps all of us at different times' (1992: 2)[2]. Most of us struggle with high levels of anxiety when we find ourselves in a state of 'not knowing'. Sinason puts this point most clearly:

> All of us, as babies, children and adults, are faced with the predicament of not knowing; we are faced with actual gaps in our knowledge; gaps in our capacity to acquire or retain kinds of knowledge; gaps in our emotional motivation that make us unable to learn certain things, quite apart from knowing what is genuinely out of our own control.
>
> (Sinason, 1992: 1)

Such a state of not knowing can, in early life, feel catastrophic. For example, the experience a baby has of a ten-minute wait for a feed can be of complete abandonment, characterised by what Winnicott (1963) describes as 'annihilatory fears'. It is only when the cognitive resources of the baby have developed, such that it has a sense of time, greater levels of self-control and the knowledge that people don't 'disappear' when out of perceptual awareness, that levels of anxiety associated with waiting become bearable.

Psychoanalytic work on human development (Klein, 1989; Wright, 1991; Winnicott, 1963; McDougal, 1974) and the processes involved in thinking (Bion, 1970, 1992) have demonstrated just how important the relationship between anxiety and thinking is. However, we need to turn to sociological work to show how cultural anxiety around that state of 'not knowing' has intensified in modern Western society. Most children growing up in Western societies are faced with a constant barrage of tests. The introduction of intelligence testing at the end of the nineteenth century occurred at the same time as the introduction of special education. The fetish around measurement and appraisal continues apace. The development of mass compulsory state education created the threat of failure for those deemed ineducable. As noted in Chapter 5, the category of 'special needs' is produced by distributing populations along a linear curve and defining those in the bottom percentiles, whatever their achievement, as 'subnormal'. The existence of categories of failure thus creates fears for everyone. For those who are firmly located in the 'successful camp', there is often a fear of being relegated to the 'failing camp'. So many of us, particularly if we have achieved the status of degree-level student or university lecturer, feel fraudulent or guilty about avoiding being discovered as stupid!

To summarise I am arguing the following:

- Psychically, we all (at an early point in life) have experience of not knowing.
- Educational culture produces failure.
- Anxiety about appearing stupid is intense in a society which places great store on 'intelligence'.

People deal with 'the sense of stupidity'[3] in different ways. Some may try to cover up areas of ignorance and difficulties in learning. Some may be dismissive about the value of certain kinds of knowledge – 'who needs maths anyway?' Some may even engage in what Sinason (1992: 2) refers to as 'defensive exaggerations' – for example, saying after an exam in which the questions turned out to be harder than expected 'I've failed'. This way, a person can nurse the secret knowledge that they have not done as badly as other people think. So one is able to reassure oneself that 'it is those who believe my lament about my disastrous exam performance that are the stupid ones!' Playing the fool is another way of dealing with the painful 'realisation that you will not be an Austin, Einstein, Madonna or Picasso' (Sinason, 1992: 20).

Either way, the sense of learning disability as the most terrible disaster and the avoidance of people with learning difficulties represent, in part, an unacknowledged identification. The more confident among us are likely to follow Confucius, who wrote, 'Shall I tell you what it is to know? To say when you know, and to say you do not when you do not, that is knowledge' (*The Analects*, quoted in Sinason, 1992).

Monstrosity

Psychoanalysis sees an appreciation of difference as one of the key emotional hurdles we all have to deal with during our early life. This point is demonstrated by Fiedler (1978), in his study of 'freaks'. He is concerned to explain the widespread awe and curiosity (although notably, not pity) felt at the sight of human 'abnormalities'. He accounts for such interest in terms of the way humans like to explore the boundaries which mark conventional categories, for example 'between male and female, sexed and sexless, animal and human, large and small, self and other, and consequently between reality and illusion, experience and fantasy, fact and myth' (Fiedler, 1978: 24).

Fascination with 'freaks' is greatest during childhood. Children love 'freaks' because they appear to establish certainty which children seek about the 'limits of our bodies and egos' (1978: 27). Thus, when pointing to the freak, children are disavowing their own bodily anxieties. The anxiety of having a body felt to be out of control is thus managed through the defence of projection. Children are obsessed with size. Giants and dwarves (and also stories such as *Alice in Wonderland* and *Jack and the Beanstalk*) exemplify concerns about scale. They can represent anxieties about growing bigger or feeling smaller. For the adolescent boy,

> his penis disconcertingly continues to rise and fall, swell and shrink – at times an imperious giant, at others a timid dwarf. For girls at puberty, the growth of breasts is similarly traumatic. It is a rare young woman who in the crisis of adolescence does not feel herself too flat-chested or too generously endowed, and in either case a Freak. ... Moreover, passing the

line of puberty means for boys and girls alike the growth of hair around the genitals more like animal fur than that on their heads. .... And when young women find what they are taught to regard as 'excess hair' ... they may doubt their femininity as well as their full humanity. .... Finally, therefore each sex tends to feel itself forever defined as freakish in relation to the other. And from our uneasiness at this, I suppose, arises the dream of androgyny.

(Fiedler, 1978: 31–2)

Hermaphrodites challenge our conviction 'that the world neatly divides into two sexes'. 'Bearded ladies' address anxieties about bodily hair and animality. 'Siamese twins' confront assumptions about separation between self and Other. Thus, the freak show enables children to project their anxieties about growing up and feeling small, developing sexual bodies, being part of mother (or inside her) and then separate from her, onto an Other. As Fiedler put it, ' "We are the Freaks," the human oddities are supposed to reassure us, from their lofty perches. "Not you. Not you!" ' (1978: 31). Fiedler thus locates the 'freakiness' not so much in the individual 'abnormal' person, but in the developmental transitions which make us all feel like freaks.

Fiedler has been accused by disability theorists such as Bogdan (1988) of naturalising 'freaks of nature'. Freaks are socially constructed rather than being essentially pathological. Bogdan argues that

Fiedler's study of 'human curiosities' ... reifies the 'freak' by taking 'it' as a constant and inevitable outpouring of basic human nature. Moreover, in his writing he slips back to treating the person exhibited as the subject of the study.

(Bogdan, 1988: 7)

Whilst this point seems justified, it does not invalidate Fiedler's important shift in focus from the disabled person to the non-disabled person's fears, fantasies and investments in disability as a category. This brings us back to the point made at the start of this book – that disability is not about disabled people, but about social and emotional relationships organised around a socially constructed difference located in particular bodies and minds.

Summary

This chapter examined some of the ways disability is produced through visual constructions. It argued that the stories contained within images of impairment both reflect and reproduce disability. This is because impairments are used in popular culture as metaphors for many (often unconscious) fears, fantasies and fetishes associated with disability. The chapter went on to identify some of the existential difficulties which many people struggle with, associated with feeling dependent, stupid and monstrous. These difficulties refer back to earlier stages in life when we were dependent, when we lacked cognitive power to make sense of the world, and when we experienced our bodies and emotions as out of control. Contemporary culture helps us to deal with these human difficulties, by locating them in particular impairments which offer non-disabled people the fantasy of being undamaged, whole and good.

Closing comments
Interdisciplinary connections, action and identity

Introduction

I had two aims in writing this book. The first was to survey the large (and rapidly growing) body of theoretical and empirical work on disability. This work reflects a very wide variety of viewpoints – all useful and indeed necessary, but all, in my view, partial and in themselves incomplete. Disability has been defined differently by a wide range of groups, each bringing their own 'models' to the problem of delineating and addressing their task. For example, civil rights activists aim to bring about the social inclusion of disabled people and have found the social model a particularly effective heuristic tool for challenging institutional and environmental barriers. Similarly, analytic therapists, concerned with helping their patients/clients become aware of unconscious fears and fantasies, focus on inter- and intra-psychic processes which generate anxieties, investments and defences in relation to the experience of disability. Finally, doctors use medical understanding to the diagnosis and treatment of 'pathological' bodies. All these models have been introduced and critically examined in this book.

My second aim has been to argue that whilst much very productive work has gone into debate the conflicts and divergent practical outcomes between each of these viewpoints, they can usefully also be understood together, as part of a wider and more holistic understanding of disability. It is important to explore the relationships between the various models and the way in which these different models have worked to constitute disability.

This concluding chapter offers some brief comments on interdisciplinarity and self-representation, as a way of moving beyond the model-making and critique discussed in the main body of this book towards new developments in theory and practice. First, I offer a short review of neuroscientific work emphasising the interrelationship between physiological constitution and experience. I identify research which shows that rather than these being separate realms, baby's brains are shaped by experiences. Having used this idea to bridge the mind–body divide, I move into the different register of politics and psychology, and identify two quite different forms of struggle towards self-representation and empowerment used by activists in the disabled people's movement: civil disobedience and the writing of accounts of experiences of disability. These activities challenge an oppressive external world and the dynamics by which this oppression comes to be internalised. As such, this part of the chapter attempts to bridge the social–psychic divide. Third, I identity some of the losses and gains which emerge out of the experience of disability, and relate complex experiences of particular impairments to key aspects of the human condition. This section explores the embodied nature of socially constructed differences. I then examine the questions of identity, wholeness and fragmentation, as central concepts for understanding both the cultural construction and unconscious fantasies of disability. I conclude by suggesting that disability is socially constructed, materially embodied, and invested with fears and fantasies. The connections between bodily, social and intra-psychic levels of experience have only just begun to be explored within neuroscience, social science and psychology. Yet such connections offer an exciting way out of the Cartesian impasse which has for so long produced a split between mind, body and society.

The physiological 'environment' and the social body

Social model theorists have rightly been highly critical of medical accounts which see disability purely in terms of physiological 'malfunctioning'. However, the social model attempt to dispense with the body and the delineation of 'impairment' as irrelevant to the understanding of disability has been criticised by a new generation of disability theorists, who have argued that we need to 'bring back' both the body and personal experience into disability theorising (Crow, 1996; Patterson, 1998).

This book has argued that such a 'return' to the body does not mean a return to biological essentialism. Chapter 5 argued that the physiological, emotional, social and cultural experiences of people

with learning difficulties and sickle cell anaemia are inextricably inter-
twined. Similarly, Chapter 6 argued that the body is a material base
for, as well as an effect of, the construction of social differences.
Patterson and Hughes (1997) have shown the extent to which what
they refer to as 'the carnal order' is informed by 'ablist' embodied
practices. Disability is not just 'out there' but also comes to be lived
and experienced physically, within particular interactional relationships. As Shilling has put it, we need to explore 'the place of the
mind in the body, rather than seeing thinking as a supra-corporeal
activity' (1997: 81).

Indeed, the body might be seen as important, not as a cause, but
rather as an *effect* of social and psychological processes. There is a
large and growing body of research which reverses conventional
(medical) assumptions about direction of causality between a
person's physiological constitution and their environment. Van der
Kolk and Greenberg (1987) and Hartman and Burgess (1993) have
demonstrated that traumatic experiences can shape the way the
brain functions (e.g. the way learning takes place). Travarthen and
Aitken (1994), Fox *et al.* (1994) and Schore (1998) have gone
further, by showing that traumatic experience actually shapes the
structure of the brain. Specifically, the baby's brain requires 'an intimate relationship [between the infant and primary care-taker] in
order to promote the development of cerebral circuits' (Schore,
1996: 62). This is because the emotions which are experienced by
the infant when interacting with his or her key attachment figure
result in the production of bio-chemicals that 'regulate the critical
growth and organisation of the developing neocortex' (Schore,
1996; 59). When an infant or child experiences repeated, prolonged
or particularly intense trauma, levels of stress hormones are altered
in such a way that damage to cells and a form of actual brain
damage can occur, in which 'states' become 'traits' (Perry, *et al.*,
1995). In other words, environmental circumstances (of a social and
interpersonal nature) can shape biological constitution. This revolutionary idea – that experience does not merely 'socialise' individuals,
but also shapes their physiological constitution – is given further
weight by research on the effect of experiences prior to birth.
Piontelli (1992) shows that events taking place in the womb and the
interaction between the mother and foetus (or between twins
foetuses) form prototype social interactions.

This research has relevance when thinking about the experiences
of many infants who have or acquire serious impairments. So many

parents of disabled children are subject to particularly high levels of stress caused by the social barriers and lack of inclusive provision for their offspring. Instead of feeling supported by the environment, such parents are often compelled to enter a battle zone in order to attain information, assistance and services for their child. Further, they are faced not with admiration for their child, but often with pity from others who see their child not as cause for celebration but for sorrow. Finally, they may be compelled to witness their child undergoing painful or uncomfortable medical and rehabilitative procedures which disrupt the parent–child relationship. Such an experience is particularly difficult when the infant is too young to understand the reason for the interventions and may experience them as an attack. Winnicott (1958) has shown that the extent to which the primary carer is valued, respected and supported (by her partner or by social networks and state institutions) plays an important role in helping her (or him) to give the infant what it needs emotionally and physiologically in order to develop. Thus many (but by no means all) disabled people experience failures not just in the social environment, but also in their emotional environment.

Those non-disabled people who have suffered similar privations (such as failures of or disruptions to empathic care) and who suffer from low self-esteem may come to identify with disabled people because of the low value accorded to them. This point is discussed in Chapter 5, which examines some of the unconscious motivations of 'compulsive carers' and other 'disability' professionals.

What is so interesting about this work is that it does not set up a competition between neuroscience, psychology and the social studies. All these studies show the importance of physiology not only as a cause but also as an effect of social and psychological events and experiences. If social model insights are combined with an analysis of psychological and physiological processes, it is possible to demonstrate a complex and contextualised picture of embodied subjects. Physiological 'damage' or social oppression can no longer be viewed as the sole causes of disability. Ultimately, the 'levels' by which we may examine disability should not be seen as competing but simply as different, multi-causal, multi-directional dimensions of understanding the relationship between the body, the psyche and the environment. As Schore puts it, we can examine human 'regulatory processes' simultaneously along several separate but interrelated dimensions, ranging from the molecular level of organization through the social and cultural levels. In fact, the adoption of this multilevel, multidisciplinary perspective is an absolute necessity for a deeper understanding of ontogeny.

(Shore, 1996: 59)

An interdisciplinary analysis exploring the connections between various levels and dimensions of experience does not invalidate the social model of disability but rather enriches it. It offers a contextualised space for exploring experiences, so that subjective aspects of disability do not need to be ghettoised into individual approaches.

The next section therefore moves from psycho-physiology to politics. This shows that responses to disablism do not just challenge social oppression but can also bring about an internal change by fostering a sense of entitlement.

Self-representation and cultural resistance

For the last twenty years, many disabled people have been engaged in active political struggles against structural barriers, attitudes and practices. Similarly, many non-disabled people have become allies in such struggles. The key feature of these struggles is that they are based on disabled people's self-representation. Oliver (1990) sees the growth in organisations of disabled people as part of a more general move from traditional party politics to a growth in 'new social movements' that are culturally oriented and tend to be focused on single issues. It is important to examine some of the ways in which disabled people and their non-disabled allies have engaged in forms of cultural resistance, and the cultural context in which such forms of resistance have become possible.

The disabled people's movement might be characterised as a 'sociocultural movement' concerned not just with obtaining civil rights, but also with obtaining what Pukulski characterises as 'cultural citizenship'. This is defined as the struggle to 're-value stigmatised identities' (Pukulski, 1996: 83) and 'redirect the claims for rights towards a new domain of cultural rights that involve the right to unhindered and legitimate representation and propagation of identities and lifestyles through information systems' (Pukulski, 1996: 74). Such a 'politics of recognition' emphasises 'not only tolerance of diverse identities but also – and increasingly – claims to endigni-fying representation' (Pukulski, 1996: 77).

One way in which disabled people have sought full 'cultural' citizenship has been through acts of civil disobedience. Until the 1990s, many acts of resistance by disabled people received little publicity (Benn, 1998; Campbell and Oliver, 1996). One such example of collective action was the protest by residents of a Cheshire home for people with physical impairments, which involved a trip to the pub in pyjamas in protest against being made 'ready for bed' prior to a change in staff shifts at 6pm[1]. The 1990s has seen a rise in the number of such acts, which have used a variety of strategies, including humour, surprise and drama, to challenge ablist environments. More recent actions by the UK Disability Action Network (DAN) have captured widespread public attention. DAN actions, which have succeeded in bringing public transport in a number of UK cities to a halt, have brought to TV screens images of disabled people in association, rather than in isolation, within public spaces, and engaged in independent activities. In this way, disabled people have succeeded in presenting subversive images of themselves as citizens in their own right, rather than as recipients of 'special' privileges extended to them out of the patronage of non-disabled people.

In the USA one important watershed in disabled people's actions was the 1988 student protest at Gallaudet University, Washington DC (Shapiro, 1994). Gallaudet is a university for Deaf people[2] and the students were protesting against the appointment of a hearing president. Whilst Howard University has had black presidents, and Wellesley College has had women presidents, Gallaudet had not, prior to 1988, had a Deaf president. The protest was difficult to control using conventional police methods, since the students' hearing impairments challenged conventional techniques of crowd control. Students set off alarms and 'a policeman tried to control the crowd by shouting directions through a megaphone. Then, realising he could not be heard', he gave up (Shapiro, 1994: 79). The protest presented a powerful visual image of hundreds of outstretched arms signing 'Deaf President Now' (Shapiro, 1994: 78). It gained national attention and the support of many local businesses and organisations, as well as widespread political support[3]. Gallaudet students were successful in securing the departure of the hearing president. Perhaps equally important, increased self-confidence and a national image of activism and resistance had been created.

Some of the campaigns by disabled people have challenged and parodied the patronising stance of non-disabled charity workers. The slogans 'Piss on Pity' and 'Blinded and Crippled by Tragic Disease'[4] present a particular 'putting-ourselves-in-the dirt humour [which] confronts the pathetic subhuman-dependency victim image of disabled people which all charity events ultimately rely on' (Hevey, 1992: 25). Such collective action breaks down the individualising experiences which are so central to the successful pathologisation of disabled people.

Aesthetic resistance

Such acts of resistance described above share one key element; they bring disabled people, *as active subjects* into a visible public arena. Disabled people's 'impairments' are neither hidden nor fetishised, but rather are *simply present*. A particularly self conscious form of visual resistance to exclusion can be found in the recent edition of the style magazine *Dazed and Confused* which contained a fashion feature entitled 'Fashion able'. Disabled people modelled clothes specially created by top fashion designers, such as Hussein Chalayan and Philip Treacy. The edition was guest edited by Alexander McQueen, dubbed the 'enfant terrible of British fashion [who]... has brought theatre and spectacle of fashion' (Hack, 1998: 8). The front cover of the magazine contains the image of the beautiful and sexy model Aimee Mullins wearing stylish 'prosthetic' lower legs. As the editorial puts it, 'the intention behind the pictures is not to be controversial. Rather this is a joyful celebration of difference' (Hack, 1998: 8). Crucially (and unusually for fashion images) the disabled models in the feature were all given a voice. In the short captions accompanying their pictures, they explained their enthusiasm for the project. Mat Fraser writes, 'the fundamental problem is that people with disabilities are invisible. We're suffering from apartheid. And most of all we're invisible in fashion and advertising... You've got to declare yourself, disabled and beautiful' (1998: 83). As Mullens writes, 'I don't want people to think I'm beautiful in spite of my disability but because of it. It's my mission to challenge people's concept of what is and isn't beautiful' (1998: 82). The feature re-addresses classical and modern conventions and iconography (for example, the image of Alison Lapper, a woman without arms, is posed in a way which is reminiscent of Venus Di Milo, yet rather than looking like a marble statue, she is covered in cubist-looking coloured shapes). Rather than attempting to make disabled people 'normal', conceptions of style and beauty are played with. We are presented with a new aesthetic which presents disabled people as *active subjects* present within the previously excluding arena of high fashion.

The personal as political: narrative accounts

In addition to collective action and aesthetic re-evaluation, there has, in the last decade, been a growth in the number of published accounts of personal experiences of disability. These have taken the form of autobiography (Hockenberry, 1996), edited collections of creative writing by and about disabled people (Keith, 1994; Saxton and Howe, 1988) and research using qualitative approaches such as open-ended interviews to narrate personal experiences (Shakespeare *et al.*, 1996; Booth and Booth, 1998).

There is some controversy in the disabled people's movement regarding the value of such accounts. There are certainly dangers in seeing narrative accounts as offering privileged access to *the* truth, when such accounts are inevitably partial. There is also a risk that a 'confessional' stance may function as a form of self-subjugation, affirming a fixed 'disabled' identity and viewed as either representing all disabled people, offering a model along the lines of 'triumphing over adversity' or reinforcing disabled people's positions as pathological objects available for voyeuristic gaze. Some social model theorists, such as Finkelstein, have described narrative accounts as diversionary and individualising, since they encourage a 'shift away from thinking about changing the real world. Finding insight in the experiences of discrimination is just a return to the old case file approach to oppression, dressed up in the social model jargon' (Finkelstein, 1996: 11).

Yet the concerns about reinforcing individualistic and pathologising images of disability are certainly not applicable to the narrative accounts referred to above, which are written within a highly theorised politicised context and which examine complex identities and experiences. Finkelstein's criticism of 'personal' accounts relies on a dualistic understanding of the relationship of the individual to society, which fails to recognise that the 'political' is embodied in the 'personal' and vice versa. Narrative accounts affirm what Williams has described as the 'multiform reality of biographical experience as it relates to both self and society' (Williams, 1984: 178).

The losses and gains associated with impairment

Narratives often demonstrate both the complex losses and difficulties, and also the unexpected gains that emerge from certain impairments and which are hard to appreciate from the 'outside'. Sacks (1987) provides many accounts of neurological defects which have advantages as well as difficult consequences. He discusses the case of 'Witty Ticcy Ray', a man with Tourette's syndrome, who was 'almost incapacitated by multiple tics of extreme violence coming in volleys every few seconds' (1987: 97). These loud, involuntary and often obscene ticks caused marital difficulties and the loss of several jobs for Ray. However, when Sacks gave Ray drugs to remove the tics, Ray lost something more than this single symptom.

> He is less sharp, less quick in repartee, no longer bubbling with witty tics. ... Most important, and disabling, because this was vital for him – as a means of support and self-expression – he found that on Haldol he was musically 'dull', average, competent, but lacking energy, enthusiasm, extravagance and joy.
>
> (Sacks, 1987: 100–1)

Eventually, Sacks and Ray found a solution which offered the best of both worlds. Ray took Haldol during the week and stopped during the weekends. As with Ray, many disabled people have mixed feelings about cure. Susan Wendell in the following passage offers a powerful expression of such ambivalence:

> I want to have more energy and less pain, and to have a more predictable body; about that there is no ambivalence. ... Yet I cannot wish that I had never contracted ME, because it has made me a different person, a person I am glad to be, would not want to have missed being, and could not imagine relinquishing, even if I were 'cured'. ... Perhaps the best summary of my attitude toward 'cure' is this: I would joyfully accept a cure, but I do not need one. If this attitude toward 'cures' were taken for granted in my society, then the search for them would not be accompanied by insulting implications, as it often is now.
>
> (Wendell, 1996: 84)

These examples show that people's experiences of illness and disability, like the human condition itself, are complex, with positive and negative aspects which give the lie, on the one hand, to fantasies of normality or even perfection, and on the other, to the denial of the significance of the impairment and associated difficulties.

Acknowledgement of both strengths and difficulties and the freedom to explore differences are central ways of understanding the complex and difficult nature of the human condition. Contextualised accounts of impairment provide a space for recognition of points of identification and difference, both within and across the dis/ability divide. Such work helps us examine the context of people's intimate experiences and the fact that what can appear to be a unique and particular situation is actually collectively shared. As Morris puts it:

> to experience disability is to experience the frailty of the human body. If we deny this we will find that our personal experience of disability will remain an isolated one; we will experience our differences as something peculiar to us as individuals – and we will commonly feel a sense of personal blame and responsibility.
>
> (Morris, 1991: 164)

Morris draws attention to the importance of engaging in the particular experiences of disabled people, not in order to pathologise these 'individuals', but rather to gain insight into general aspects of the human condition. Narrative takes us away from abstract theorising, and brings us closer to the messy and complex embodied realities of lives. It demonstrates that experiences of disability, like experiences of 'ability', tend to be ambivalent, conflicting and changing. Moreover, such complexity means that disability cannot be reduced to that which is measurable and classifiable. Narratives challenge crude social psychological and experimental research which tries to discover a singular truth. It can also challenge one-dimensional personal tragedy stories or those attempts to counter personal tragedy theory by denying the significance of impairment. Rather than silencing such narratives of impairment through what French has described as 'polite reminders' [by orthodox social model theorists] 'that I am talking about "impairment" not "disability", or suggesting that the problems I describe have nothing to do with lack of sight but do indeed lie "out there" in the physical and social environment' (1994: 19), narrative offers a space to explore the meanings of impairment and other differences.

Identity and fragmentation

The sense of what constitutes a whole body was disrupted in the First World War, when young men underwent amputations on a scale hitherto unknown (Bourke, 1996). As the work of Haraway (1991) has shown, understandings of bodily boundaries underwent further change with the development of biotechnologies after the Second World War. Twentieth-century uncertainty about the unified individual subject is reflected not just in the social sciences but also in art. Cubism, Surrealism and contemporary art demonstrate, in different ways, concerns and anxieties about the 'unified' Cartesian subject. In what some commentators refer to as 'post-modern' society, identities have become increasingly contingent. This is in part due to globalisation, which has loosened the link between identity, cultural specificity and location. More and more people experience separation from their geographical and cultural 'origins' and 'ethnic' identities have become increasingly indeterminate. Similarly, sexual orientation and identity have become increasingly open and negotiable. Alongside increasing cultural and sexual hybridity, dis/abled identities seem to be becoming increasingly contested and negotiable. Cooper (1997) struggles with the question of whether 'a fat woman can call herself disabled'. Chapters 1 and 6 underline the contingency of the status 'disabled' and the status 'non-disabled'. Changing technologies, administrative and cultural practices, demographics and relationships transform the perception and treatment of embodied differences. The twenty-first century is likely to see changes in social structure, practices and identities, perhaps at a faster rate than those witnessed over the last few decades.

The sharp division between the 'whole' and the 'impaired is thus not a permanent dividing line, but rather a continuum through which a large proportion of the population will travel. It has been a central concern of this book to illustrate how society defines and delineates disability. This process of defining disability is undertaken for a wide range of administrative and cultural purposes. At the same time this book has emphasised the way in which disabled people have begun to play a major part in defining themselves, and the way in which the nature of our understanding of disability is affected by the interaction of these disparate viewpoints and interests.

The rise of disabled people's increasingly assertive consciousness and activism is, of course, one element in the emergence of an increasingly complex and self-aware Western culture that is likely to dominate the thinking and attitudes of the twenty-first century. A growing pluralism – in terms of ethnicity, gender and sexual orientation – will form the context in which the debate about the 'normal' and the 'abnormal', the 'whole' and the 'impaired', the 'abled and the 'disabled' will take place. It has been the purpose of this book to make a contribution to that debate by illustrating some of the current controversies and dilemmas, and by setting out some of the theoretical issues raised.

The social construction of disability

This book has argued that disability is not an essential quality, but rather that it is a social construction. The category 'disability' measures individual citizens according to criteria that establish their fitness for work, entitlement to certain 'services' and 'benefits', and inclusion within 'mainstream' society. The notion of who fits into the category of 'able-bodied' and 'disabled' changes depending on a wide range of technological, organisational and cultural factors. Whether disability is constituted between the charity donor and the 'beneficiary', the 'beauty' and the 'freak', or the professional and the service user, disability can only ever be a relational concept. The ability/disability binary is thus produced through a range of structures (such as the built environment and the hierarchical organisation of the medical profession), practices (such as the professional treatment of disabled people) and symbols (within the media, literature and art), which maintain, justify and reproduce disability.

Disability and ability are not fixed states, but rather are contingent positions. The social construction and psychological reproduction of disability both oppress those constituted as disabled and regulate those constituted as able. Both categories of disability and ability require work in order to be maintained.

Much of the work of Disability Studies scholars has been to make visible those normally hidden processes and structures which produce disability and 'normality'. The concern is not just with how the person 'is', but rather how they 'come to be' in specific socio-cultural contexts. Disability Studies as a discipline has been concerned to denaturalise assumptions about what 'disability' and 'ability' is. In so doing, it demonstrates that things need not be as they currently are.

In the UK, the discipline has broadly focused on disabling social structures and policies (Shakespeare, 1998), whilst in the USA, the discipline has, to a greater extent, addressed the historical, cultural and social-psychological conditions producing disability (Davis, 1997). In this book, I have attempted to bring together these two approaches, whilst adding a third perspective, which looks not just at the construction of disability, but at the *embodied* people who occupy positions, as disabled and non-disabled, and who invest these positions with *aesthetic and moral values, fears* and *fantasies*. Many of these psychological investments are unconscious.

In order to explore some of these 'unspeakable' and 'unthinkable' experiences of disability, I have examined widespread anxieties, for example concerning the sense of 'stupidity', 'dependency' and 'monstrosity' experienced by infants and children when confronted with the developmental tasks associated with learning, separating and becoming responsible and sexual adults in contemporary Western society. When these tasks are experienced as unmanageable they are more likely to be disavowed. Disabled people, who have been socially constituted as 'damaged' have become, in contemporary society, convenient repositories for these affects. Such projections can lead non-disabled people to fear or care for disabled people, as ways of avoiding getting away from or looking after parts of their self which have been disowned.

I have also examined some of the ways in which projections of damage, fragmentation and lack can be internalised by disabled people. When such internalised oppression is unconscious, the sense of shame may be defended against using a range of defence mechanisms which help disabled people to survive (but not necessarily resist or free themselves from) denigrating projections. Finally, I have looked at some of the ways in which disabled people have begun to successfully resist disablist projections, through collective political action, through asserting new aesthetic images of disability and through presenting narrative accounts of their experiences. Self-representation which both engages with and disrupts disablist culture thus offers a space for new identities. What has been constituted as disability and is subsequently hidden, displayed or excluded can perhaps begin to be respected and included within a transformed social and cultural environment.

This work of bringing together different 'models' of disability represents an attempt to foster new collaboration, across disciplines and between people in different structural locations and with different identities on the dis/ability continuum, with a view to disrupting disablist oppression and undermining hierarchical regulatory practice.

Notes

Introduction

1 Wolfensberger uses the term 'deathmaking' to refer to 'any action or pattern of actions which either directly or indirectly bring about, or hasten, the death of a person, group or class' (Wolfensberger, 1994: 290).

Chapter I

1 Coined by Daniel Marks.
2 Generally, however, this book uses the term 'non-disabled', since it is less burdened with powerful emotional overtones which raise the temperature in an already heated debate. A further discussion of the complex terminology wars will be offered in Chapter 7.
3 Klein developed 'object relations theory' which examines relations not just between people, but also between parts of people (e.g. the way a baby recognises its mother's smell, or her breast or experiences her as good or hateful, before it is able to recognise her as a whole person). The term 'objects' rather than 'people' is useful, since we do not always relate to a whole person. 'Part-object' thinking may involve fetishising one aspect of a person and seeing that part as standing for the whole. Such thinking forms a central feature involved in stereotyping 'Others' – for example, by reducing the disabled person to their impairment.
4 See textbooks such as Sander *et al* (1997), Bateman and Holmes (1995), Gomez (1997) or dictionaries such as Laplanche and Pontalis (1988), Ryecroft, (1972), Hinshelwood (1998), Abrams (1996), Fenichel (1990) and Evans (1997) for a more detailed introductory outline to psychoanalytic concepts.
5 Indeed, the term 'trauma', as it is used in psychoanalysis, means a 'shocking experience that breaks through the protective shield of the psyche and cannot be processed' (Sinason, 1992: 327).
6 What Skynner describes as the 'myth of altruism' will be discussed further in Chapter 5.

Chapter 2

1 The term 'infanticidal introject' was coined by Brett Khar at the Mental Handicap Workshop at the Tavistock clinic. In psychoanalytic terminology an introject is the mirror image of the term 'projection' discussed in the Introduction.
2 This point is discussed further in Chapter 8, when I discuss non-disabled people's disavowal of feelings of stupidity.
3 Personal communication, December 1998.

Chapter 3

1 This term was coined by Wendell (1996) in her excellent philosophical exploration of personal experiences of disability.
2 See Malan's (1986) triangular model of the 'victim, rescuer and persecutor'.
3 Later on in the chapter I outline the contribution psychoanalysis has made to exploring the dehumanising, fetishising and pacifying aspects of modern medical care.
4 In the Conclusion I identify some of the ways in which 'symptoms' of pathology are used in a productive, creative and life-enhancing way.
5 From the organisation DAD discussed further in Chapter 6.
6 A term used by Winnicott (1960) to refer to the state of integration felt by an infant when provided with a secure environment.
7 This relational perspective is in marked contrast with the individualist orientation of Descartes' famous dictum, 'I think, therefore I am.'
8 The dynamics of performing difference are discussed in Chapter 8.

Chapter 5

1 This is a senior position which enables the therapist to take on trainee therapists as their clients.
2 That is, responses which involve transferring feelings from a previous period of life onto current relationships. As Laplanche and Pontalis put it, 'Infantile prototypes can thus re-emerge and are experienced with a strong sensation of immediacy' (1988: 455).
3 Chapter 6 identifies some of the differences between disabled people.
4 Many of the residents in the unit had several convictions for violent and sexual offences.
5 Parker *et al.* (1995) offer a long list of organisations which contain a mix of professionals, allies and survivors of the mental health system, who work collaboratively to bring about change.

Chapter 6

1 This point does not, however mean that we should use life-cycle models reductively in classifying disabled people according to their age and impairment, in the way that some theorists have done.

2 In the Conclusion I discuss some of the strategies used by disabled people to resist bodily regulations.
3 Corrine Kirschner used this term in a conversation in 1996.
4 Thanks to Anna Ravetz for offering this example of her work (November 1988).

Chapter 7

1 By the twentieth century, the extent to which confinement was necessary to discipline those identified as mad was reduced, because of the introduction of pharmacological treatments, psychosurgery and electric shock 'therapy'.

Chapter 8

1 I have been asked by the charity in question to make no reference to its name when using this picture because it no longer wishes to be associated with the image in question.
2 Chapter 3 addresses the way in which people with learning difficulties are particularly vulnerable to 'secondary handicaps'.
3 This phrase is taken from the title of Sinason (1992), Chapter 2.

Conclusion

1 Thanks to Jane Campbell for sharing this story.
2 When a capital initial is used in 'Deaf', the word refers to a community of sign language users, rather than to those people who have a hearing impairment.
3 Including that of Senator Bob Dole and Vice President George Bush, who were battling for the Republican presidential nomination.
4 A poster used by equality trainer Mike Higgins in a protest against charity.

Bibliography

Ablon, J. (1984) *Little People in America: The Social Dimension of Dwarfism*, New York: Praeger.

—— (1990) 'Ambiguity and Difference: Families with Dwarf Children', *Social Science and Medicine*, 30(8), 879–87.

Abrams, J. (1996) *The Language of Winnicott: A Dictionary of Winnicott's Use of Words*, London: Karnac Books.

Albrecht, G. (1992) *The Disability Business: Rehabilitation in America*, London: Sage Library of Social Research, 190.

Aldridge, J. and Becker, S. (1994) *My Child My Carer*, Department of Social Sciences, Loughborough: Loughborough University.

Armstrong, D. (1983) *The Political Anatomy of the Human Body: Medical Knowledge in Britain in the Twentieth Century*, Cambridge: Cambridge University Press.

Asche, A. (1988) 'Reproductive Technologies and Disability', in S. Cohen and N. Taub (eds) *Reproductive Laws for the 1990's*, Clifton, NJ: Humana Press.

Austin, J. (1962) *How to Do Things With Words*, London: Oxford University Press.

Barnes, C. (1990) *Cabbage Syndrome: The Social Construction of Dependency*, London: Tavistock Press.

—— (1992) *Disabling Imagery and the Media*, Halifax: BCODP and Ryburn Publishing.

—— (1994) *Disabled People in Britain and Discrimination: A Case for Anti-Discrimination Legislation*, London: Hurst and Company in Association with BCODP.

—— (1996) 'The Social Model: Myths and Misconceptions', *Coalition*, August: 27–35.

Barnes, C. and Mercer, G. (eds) (1996) *Exploring the Divide: Illness and Disability*, Leeds: The Disability Press.

Barnes, M. (1997) *Care, Communities and Citizens*, London: Longman.

Barton, L. and Clough, P. (eds) (1995) *Making Difficulties: Research and the Construction of Special Educational Needs*, London: Paul Chapman Publishing.

Bateman, A. and Holmes, J. (1995) *Introduction to Psychoanalysis: Contemporary Theory and Practice*, London: Routledge.

Baynton, D.C. (1996) *Forbidden Signs: American Culture and the Campaign Against Sign Language*, Chicago: Chicago University Press.

Begum, N. (1992) 'Disabled Women and the Feminist Agenda', *Feminist Review*, 40: 3–6.

—— (1996) 'Doctor, Doctor... Disabled Women's Experiences of General Practitioners', in J. Morris (ed.) *Encounters with Strangers*.

Begum, N., Hill, M. and Stevens, A. (eds) (1994) *Reflections: The Views of Black Disabled People on their Lives and Community Care*, London: CCETSW.

Bendelow, G. and Williams, S. (1995) 'Transcending the Dualisms: Towards a Sociology of Pain', *Sociology of Health and Illness*, 17: 139–65.

Benn, M. (1998) 'A Very Able Body', *The Guardian*, 15 December: 4–5.

Beresford, P. and Campbell, J. (1994) 'Disabled People, Service Users, User Involvement and Representation', *Disability and Society*, 9(3): 315–26.

Bilton, T., Bonnet, L., Jones, P., Skinner, D., Stanworth, M. and Webster, A. (1996) *Introductory Sociology*, 3rd edn, London: Macmillan.

Bion, W.R. (1961) *Experiences in Groups and Other Papers*, London: Tavistock Publications Limited.

—— (1967) 'A Theory of Thinking', in *Second Thoughts*, New York: Jason Aronson.

—— (1970) *Attention and Interpretation*, London: Tavistock.

—— (1992) *Cogitations*, London: Karnac.

Bliss, S. (1994) 'Perfection or Preconception – Some Thoughts on Reactions to Disability in the Therapist', *British Journal of Psychotherapy*, 11(1): 115–19.

Bogdan, R. (1988) *Freak Show: Presenting Human Oddities for Amusement and Profit*, Chicago: University of Chicago Press.

Bollas, C. (1987) *The Shadow of the Object: Psychoanalysis of the Unthought Known*, London: Free Association Books.

Booth, T. and Booth, W. (1998) *Growing Up With Parents Who Have Learning Difficulties*, London: Routledge.

Bordo, S. (1993) 'Feminism, Foucault and the Politics of the Body', in C. Ramazanoglu (ed.) *Up Against Foucault: Explorations of Some Tensions Between Foucault and Feminism*, London: Routledge.

Bott Spillius, E. (1990) Asylum and Society, in E. Trist and H. Murray (eds) *The Social Engagement of Social Science*, vol. 1, *The Social-Psychological Perspective*, London: Free Association Books.

Bourdieu, P. (1992) *Invitation to Reflexive Sociology*, Chicago: Chicago University Press.

Bourke, J. (1996) *Dismembering the Male: Men's Bodies, Britain and the Great War*, London: Reaktion Books.

Bowlby, J. (1973) *Attachment and Loss*, vol. 2, *Separation*, New York: Basic Books.

Bowman, N. (1986) 'Maladjustment: A History of the Category', in W. Swann (ed.) *The Practice of Special Education*.

Bowron, R. (ed.) (1998) 'Worlds of Difference Supplement', *BBC World Service*, London: BBC.

Broom, B. (1997) *Somatic Illness: The Patient's Other Story*, London: Free Association Books.

Brown, H. and Turk, V. (1992) 'Defining Sexual Abuse as it Effects Adults with Learning Disabilities', *Mental Handicap*, 20: 44–5.

Bunton, R. and Burrows, R. (1995) 'Consumption and Health in the "Epidemiological" Clinic of Late Modern Medicine', in R. Bunton, S. Nettleton and R. Burrows (eds) *The Sociology of Health Promotion: Critical Analyses of Consumption, Lifestyle and Risk*, London: Routledge.

Burr, V. (1995) *An Introduction to Social Constructionism*, London: Routledge.

Bury, M. (1996) 'Defining and Researching Disability: Issues at Stake', in C. Barnes and G. Mercer (eds) *Exploring the Divide*.

Butler, J. (1993) *Bodies That Matter: On the Discursive Limits of 'Sex'*, London: Routledge.

Butterfield, H. (1931) *The Whig Interpretation of History*, London: Bell and Sons.

Campbell, J. and Oliver, M. (1996) *Disability Politics*, London: Routledge.

Changing Faces (1998), a documentary about cosmetic surgery for people with Down's syndrome, directed by N. Finnis for Yorkshire TV, 24 November.

Collier, P. (1987) The Educational Needs of Girls, unpublished discussion document for Manchester Education Committee.

Cooper, C. (1997) 'Can a Fat Woman Call Herself Disabled?', *Disability and Society*, 12(1): 31–41.

Corbett, A., Cottis, T. and Morris, S. (1996) *Witnessing, Nurturing, Protesting: Therapeutic Responses to Sexual Abuse of People with Learning Disabilities*, London: David Fulton.

Corbett, J. (1994) 'A Proud Label: Exploring the Relationship Between Disability Politics and Gay Pride', *Disability and Society*, 19(3).

Croll, P., Moser, D. and Wright, J. (1984) 'Children with "Learning Difficulties" and Assessment in the Junior Classroom', in P. Broadfoot (ed.) *Selection, Certification and Control: Social Issues in Educational Assessment*, London: The Falmer Press.

Crossley, N. (1993) 'The Politics of Gaze: Between Foucault and Merleau-Ponty', *Human Studies*, 16: 399–41.

—— (1995) 'Merleau-Ponty, the Elusive Body and Carnal Sociology', *Body and Society*, 1(1): 43–63.

Crow, L. (1996) 'Including All of Our Lives: Renewing the Social Model of Disabilty', in C. Barnes and G. Mercer (eds) *Exploring the Divide.*

Csordas, T. (1994) *Embodiment and Experience: The Existential Ground of Culture and Self*, Cambridge: Cambridge University Press.

Cumberbatch, G. and Negrine, R. (1992) *Images of Disability on Television*, London: Routledge.

Curt, B.C. (1994) *Textuality and Tectonics: Troubling Social and Psychological Science*, Buckingham: Open University Press.

Darke, P.A. (1994) 'The Elephant Man (David Lynch, EMI Films, 1980): An Analysis From a Disabled Perspective', *Disability and Society*, 9(3): 327–42.

—— (1997) 'Film and Disability: From Polemical Theory to Defining Analysis', *Book Four: Discursive Practices*, MA Disability Studies Distance Learning Course, Centre for Psychotherapeutic Studies, Sheffield University.

Davis, K. (1994) 'The Crafting of Good Clients', in J. Swain *et al.* (eds), *Disabling Barriers.*

Davis, L. (1995) *Enforcing Normalcy: Disability, Deafness, and the Body*, New York: Verso

—— (1997) (ed.) *The Disability Studies Reader*, London: Routledge.

Dazed and Confused (1998) 'Fashion able', 46.

De Jong, G. (1993) 'Health Care Reform and Disability: Affirming Our Commitment to Community', *Arch. Phys. Medical Rehabilitation*, 74, October: 1017–24.

Diseker, R.A. and Michielutte, R. (1981) 'An Analysis of Empathy in Medical Students Before and Following Clinical Experience', *Journal of Medical Education*, 56: 1004–10.

Donzelot, J. (1980) *The Policing of Families: Welfare Versus the State*, London: Hutchinson.

Douglas, M. (1991 [1966]) *Purity and Danger: An Analysis of the Concepts of Pollution and Taboo*, London: Routledge.

Doyal, L. and Gough, I. (1991) *A Theory of Human Need*, Basingstoke: Macmillan.

Driedger, D. (1989) *The Last Civil Rights Movement*, London: Hurst.

Dutton, K.R. (1995) *The Perfectible Body: The Western Ideal of Physical Development*, London: Cassell.

Dyson, S. (1986) (1996) 'Deconstructing Genetic Counselling: The Case of Haemoglobinopathy Counsellors in the UK', paper presented to *Deconstructing Professions: Professional Identity and Professional Order in Comparative Context*, Biannual International Conference, Spain, 25–6 April.

Edgerton, R.B. (1967) *The Cloak of Competence: Stigma in the Lives of the Mentally Retarded*, Berkeley and Los Angeles: University of California Press.

Edwards, D., Ashmore, M. and Potter, J. (1995) 'Death and Furniture: The Rhetoric, Politics and Theology of Bottom-Line Arguments Against Relativism', *History of the Human Sciences*, 8(2): 25–49.

Elias, N. (1978)*The Civilizing Process*, vol. 1, *The History of Manners*, New York: Pantheon Books.

—— (1983) *The Court Society*, Oxford: Basil Blackwell.

Engels, F. (1958) *The Condition of the Working Class in England*, translated by W.O.

Englehardt Jr, H.T. (1986) *The Foundations of Bioethics*, Oxford: Oxford University Press.

Erskine, A. and Judd, D. (eds) (1994) *The Imaginative Body: Psychodynamic Therapy in Health Care*, London: Whurr.

Evans, D. (1997) *An Introductory Dictionary of Lacanian Psychoanalysis*, London: Routledge.

Evans, J. (1988) 'The Iron Cage', *Ten 8 Photographic Magazine*, 29.

—— (1992) 'Infantilism, Projection and Naturalism in the Construction of Mental Disablement', in D. Hevey, *The Creatures Time Forgot*.

Evans-Pritchard, E.E. (1940) *The Nuer*, Oxford, Oxford University Press.

Farqueson, G. (1999) 'Institutional Dynamics', lecture to MA Disability Studies Course, Centre for Psychotherapeutic Studies, Sheffield University, 26 March.

Felce, D. and Emerson, E. (1996) 'Challenging Behaviour and the Need for Evidence-Based Services', *Journal of Applied Research in Intellectual Disabilities*, 9(3).

Fenichel, O. (1990) *The Psychoanalytic Theory of Neurosis*, London: Routledge.

Fernando, S. (1993) 'Psychiatry and Racism', *Changes: An International Journal of Psychology and Psychotherapy*, 10: 46–58.

Fiedler, L.A. (1978) *Freaks: Myths and Images of the Secret Self*, London: Penguin.

Finkelstein, V. (1980) *Attitudes and Disabled People: Issues for Discussion*, New York: World Rehabilitation Fund.

—— (1996) 'The Disability Movement Has Run Out of Steam', *Disability Now*, February: 11.

Fonagy, P. and Target, M. (1998) 'An Interpersonal View of the Infant', in A. Hurry (ed.) *Psychoanalysis and Developmental Theory*.

Ford, P. (1997) 'The Life of the Elephant Man', in *QED: The True Story of the Elephant Man*, London: BBC Learning Support.

Ford, P. and Howell, D. (1992) *The History of the Elephant Man*, London: Penguin.

Foucault, M. (1976) *Birth of the Clinic: An Archaeology of Medical Perception*, London: Tavistock.

—— (1977) *Discipline and Punish: The Birth of the Prison*, translated by Alan Sheridan, New York: Pantheon.

——— (1995) *Madness and Civilization: A History of Insanity in the Age of Reason*, London: Routledge.

Fox, N., Calkins, S. and Bell, M.A. (1994) 'Neural Plasticity and Development in the First Two Years of Life: Evidence for Cognitive and Socioemotional Domains of Research', *Development and Psychopathology*, 6: 677–96.

Frank, A.W. (1991) 'From Sick Role to Health Role: Deconstructing Parsons', in R. Robertson and B.S. Turner (eds) *Talcott Parsons: Theorist of Modernity*, London: Sage.

French, S. (1994) 'Disability, Impairment of Something in Between', in J. Swain *et al.* (eds) *Disabling Barriers.*

——— (1996) 'Simulation Exercises in Disability Awareness Training: a Critique', in G. Hales (ed.) *Beyond Disability.*

——— (1996a) 'The Attitudes of Health Professionals Towards Disabled People', in G. Hales (ed.) *Beyond Disability.*

Freud, S. (1914) *Remembering, Repeating the Working Through, The Standard Edition of the Complete Psychological Works of Sigmund Freud*, vol. 12, London: The Hogarth Press.

——— (1933) *New Introductory Lectures on Psycho-Analysis*, in *Standard Edition*, vol. 22.

——— (1973) 'Fixation – The Unconscious', in *Introductory Lectures on Psychoanalysis*, The Pelican Freud Library, vol. 1, London: Pelican.

Frosh, S. (1997) *For and Against Psychoanalysis*, London: Routledge.

Fuss, D. (1989) *Essentially Speaking: Feminism, Nature and Difference*, London: Routledge.

Gallagher, H.G. (1985) *FDR's Splendid Deception*, New York: Dodd, Mead and Company.

——— (1990) *By Trust Betrayed: Patients and Physicians in the Third Reich*, London: Henry Hold.

Garkfinkel, H. (1967) *Studies in Ethnomethodology*, Englewood Cliffs: Prentice Hall.

Garland Thompson, R. (ed.) (1996) *Freakery: Cultural Spectacles of the Extraordinary Body*, New York: New York University Press.

——— (1997) *Extraordinary Bodies: Figuring Physical Disability in American Culture and Literature*, London: Routledge.

Gartner, A. and Joe, T. (1987) *Images of The Disabled, Disabling Images*, New York: Praeger.

Gatens, M. (1993) *Imaginary Bodies: Ethics, Power and Corporeality*, London: Routledge.

Gerber, D. (1996) 'Volition and Valorisation: The "Careers" of People Exhibited in Freak Shows', in R. Garland Thompson (ed.) *Freakery.*

Gerhardt, U. (1989) *Ideas about Illness: An Intellectual and Political History of Medical Sociology*, London: Macmillan.

Gilman, S.L. (1988) *Disease and Regeneration*, New York: Cornell.

Glover, J. (1977) *Causing Death and Saving Lives*, Harmondsworth: Penguin.

—— (1990) *Causing Death and Saving Lives*, London: Penguin.

Goffman, I. (1961) *Asylums: Essays on the Social Situation of Mental Patients and Other Inmates*, London: Pelican.

—— (1963) *Stigma: Notes on the Management of Spoiled Identity*, London: Penguin.

Goldberg, D. and Huxley, P. (1992) *Common Mental Disorders: a Bio-Social Model*, London: Tavistock and Routledge.

Gomez, L. (1997) *An Introduction to Object Relations*, London: Free Association Books.

Goode, D. (1994) *A World Without Words: The Social Construction of Children Born Deaf and Blind*, Philadelphia: Temple University Press.

Gooding, C. (1995) *A Guide to the Disability Discrimination Act*, London: Blackstone Press.

Grealy, L. (1994) *Autobiography of a Face*, Boston and New York: Houghton Mifflin.

Groce, N. (1985) *Everyone Here Spoke Sign Language: Heredity Deafness on Martha's Vineyard*, London: Harvard University Press.

—— (1992) ' "The Town Fool": An Oral History of a Mentally Retarded Individual in a Small Town Society', in P.M. Ferguson, D.L. Ferguson and S.J. Taylor (eds) *Interpreting Disability: A Qualitative Reader*, New York: Teachers College Press.

Gullo, J. (1991) 'Oscaring the Handicaps', *Premier*, April: 36

Gwynne, G. and Miller, E. (1972) *A Life Apart*, London: Tavistock Press.

Hack, J. (1998) 'From the Editor', *Dazed and Confused*, 46.

Hales, G. (1996) *Beyond Disability: Towards an Enabling Society*, London: Sage in association with the Open University Press.

Hall, S. (1990) 'Cultural Identity and Diaspora', in J. Rutherford (ed.) *Identity, Community, Culture, Difference*, London: Lawrence and Wishart.

—— (1997) 'The Work of Representation', in *Representation: Cultural Representations and Signifying Practices*, London: Sage in association with the Open University Press.

Haraway, D.J. (1991) 'A Cyborg Manifesto: Science, Technology and Socialist-Feminism in the Late Twentieth Century', in *Simions, Cyborgs and Women: The Reinvention of Nature*, London: Free Association Books.

—— (1994) 'A Game of Cat's Cradle: Science Studies, Feminist Theory, Cultural Studies', *Configurations*, 1: 59–71.

Hartman, C. and Burgess, A. (1993) 'Information Processing of Trauma', *Child Abuse and Neglect*, 17: 47–8.

Hasler, F. (1993) 'Developments in the Disabled People's Movement', in J. Swain *et al.* (eds) *Disabling Barriers*.

Hattersley, P., Duke, N. Mirfin, C. and Roe, A. (1992) *Disability and Dedication: Help, Advice, Awareness, Access*, flyer, Sheffield: DAD.

Hegarty, S., Pocklington, K. and Lucas, D. (1981) *Educating Pupils with Special Needs in Ordinary Schools*, Windsor: Nfer-Nelson.

Hevey, D. (1992) *The Creatures Time Forgot: Photography and Disability Imagery*, London: Routledge.

Hill, D. (1983) *The Politics of Schizophrenia: Psychiatric Oppression in the United States*, London: University Press of America.

Hinshelwood, R.D. (1998) *A Dictionary of Kleinian Thought*, London: Free Association Books.

Hockenberry, J. (1996) *Declarations of Independence: War Zones and Wheelchairs*, London: Viking.

Hoggett, P. (1992) *Partisans in an Uncertain World: The Psychoanalysis of Engagement*, London: Free Association Books.

Holmes, J. (1998) 'The Changing Aims of Psychoanalytic Psychotherapy: an Integrative Perspective', *The International Journal of Psycho-Analysis*, 79(2), April.

Hubbard, R. (1997) 'Abortion and Disability: Who Should and Should Not Inhabit the World', in L. Davis (ed.) *The Disability Studies Reader*.

Hughes, B. and Paterson, K. (1997) 'The Social Model of Disability and the Disappearing Body: Towards a Sociology of Impairment', *Disability and Society*, 12 (3): 325–40.

Hugman, R. (1991) *Power in Caring Professions*, London: Macmillan.

Hull, J. (1997) *On Sight and Insight: A Journey into the World of Blindness*, Oxford: One World.

Hunt, P. (1966) 'A Critical Condition', in *Stigma: The Experience of Disability*, London: Geoffrey Chapman.

—— (1981) 'Settling Accounts with the Parasite People', *Disability Challenge*, 1, London: UPIAS.

Hunt, S. and Symonds, A. (1995) *The Social Meaning of Midwifery*, London: Macmillan.

Hurry, A. (ed.) *Psychoanalysis and Developmental Theory*, London: Karnac.

Illich, I. (1977) *Limits of Medicine, Medical Nemesis: The Expropriation of Health*, Harmondsworth: Penguin.

Imrie, R. (1996) *Disability and the City: International Perspectives*, London: Paul Chapman Publishing.

Ingstad, B. and Whyte, S.R. (1995) *Disability and Culture*, London: University of California Press.

Jenks, C. (1998) (ed.) *Core Sociological Dichotomies*, London: Sage.

Jolley, M. and Perry, A. (1996) 'Social Class Stratification and Health Inequality', in A. Perry (ed.) *Sociology: Insights in Health Care*, London: Arnold Press.

Kanner, L. (1942) 'Exoneration of the Feebleminded', *American Journal of Psychiatry*, 99(1): 17–22.

Karen, R. (1998) *Becoming Attached: First Relationships and How They Shape Our Capacity to Love*, Oxford: Oxford University Press.

Keith, L. (1994) *Mustn't Grumble: Writings by Disabled Women*, London: The Women's Press.

Keith, L. and Morris, J. (1996) 'A Disability Rights Perspective on the "Children as Carers" Debate', in J. Morris (ed.) *Encounters with Strangers*.

Kennedy, F. (1942) 'The Problem of Social Control of the Congenital Defective – Education, Sterilization, Euthanasia', *American Journal of Psychiatry*, Vol. 99 (1), 13–16.

Kennedy, M. (1996) 'Sexual Abuse and Disabled Children', in J. Morris (ed.) *Encounters with Strangers*.

Kitzinger, C. (1987) *The Social Construction of Lesbianism*, London: Sage.

Kitzinger, J. (1990) 'Who Are You Kidding? Children, Power and the Struggle Against Sexual Abuse', in A. James and A. Prout (eds) *Constructing and Reconstructing Childhood*, London: The Falmer Press.

Klatt, H.J. (1991) 'Learning Disabilities: A Questionable Construct', in *Educational Theory*, 41(1), Winter: 34–40.

Klein, M. (1952) 'Some Theoretical Conclusions Regarding the Emotional Life of the Infant', *Developments*, 202.

—— (1989) *Narrative of a Child Analysis*, London: Virago Press.

Klobas, L.E. (1988) *Disability Drama in Television and Film*, Jefferson: McFarland and Company.

Kohon, G. (1986) *The British School of Psychoanalysis: The Independent Tradition*, London: Free Association Books.

Kovel, J. (1988) *White Racism*, London: Free Association Books.

Kraemer, S. (1994) ' "The Body Goes Mad": Hospital Liaison Psychiatry in Sickle-Cell Disease', in A. Erskine and D. Judd (eds) *The Imaginative Body*.

Kriegel, L. (1969) 'Uncle Tom and Tiny Tim: Some Reflections on the Cripple as Negro', *The American Scholar*, 38(3), Summer: 412–30.

Lacan, J. (1977) *Ecrits: A Selection*, London: Tavistock.

Laing, R.D. and Esterson, A. (1964) *Sanity, Madness and the Family: Families of Schizophrenics*, London: Tavistock.

Laplanche, J. and Pontalis, J.B. (1988) *The Language of Psychoanalysis*, London: Karnac.

Lawton, H. (1982) 'The Myth of Altruism', *Journal of Psychohistory*, 9(3): 265–308.

Leder, D. (1990) *The Absent Body*, Chicago: University of Chicago Press.

Lenny, J. (1994) 'Do Disabled People Need Counselling?', in J. Swain *et al.* (eds) *Disabling Barriers*.

Lifton, R.J. (1986) *The Nazi Doctors: Medical Killing and the Psychology of Genocide*, London: Papermac.

Linton, S. (1998) 'Disability Studies/Not Disability Studies', *Disability and Society*, 13(4), September.

Longmore, P. (1987) 'Screening Stereotypes: Images of Disabled People in Television and Motion Pictures', in A. Gartner and T. Joe (eds) *Images of The Disabled*, pp. 65–78

Lupton, D. (1995) *The Imperative of Health: Public Health and the Regulated Body*, London: Sage.

—— (1997) 'Foucault and the Medicalisation Critique', in *Foucault, Medicine and Health*, London: Routledge, pp .94–110.

Lysons, K. (1996) *Understanding Hearing Loss*, London: Jessica Kingsley.

McDermot, J.J. (1986) *Streams of Experience: Reflections in the History and Philosophy of American Culture*, Amherst: University of Massachusetts Press.

McDonagh, P. (1995) 'What's Eating the Community Living Movement: Movies, Autism and 'Traditional Values', paper given at *Thisability*, University of Michigan, Saturday 20 May.

McDougal, J. (1974) 'The Psychosoma and the Psychoanalytic Process', *International Review of Psycho-Analysis*, 1: 437–59.

McQueen, A. (1998) (guest editor) 'Access-Able', *Dazed and Confused*, 46, 68–83.

Mailhot, A. (1995) 'Any Choice You Want: As Long As It's Death', *The Disability Rag and ReSource*, January/February.

Mairs, N. (1986) 'On Being a Cripple', *Plaintexts: Essays*, 9–20, Tuscon: University of Arizona Press.

Malan, D. (1986) *Individual Psychotherapy and the Science of Psychodynamics*, London: Butterworth.

Mallory, B.L., Nichols, R.W., Charlton, J.I. and Marfo, K. (1993) *Traditional and Changing Views of Disability in Developing Societies: Causes and Consequences, Cautions*, Monograph no. 53), University of New Hampshire: International Exchange of Experts and Information in Rehabilitation.

Marker, R. (1995) 'From Michigan Van to Oregon Trail', *The Disability Rag and ReSource*, January/February.

Marks, D. (1993) 'Discourse Analysis and Education Case Conferences', Ph.D. Thesis, Manchester Metropolitan University.

—— (1996a) 'Able-Bodied Dilemmas in Teaching Disability Studies', *Feminism and Psychology*, 6 (1), February: 69–74.

—— (1996b) 'The Crafting of Care: Rationality, Gender and Social Relations in Educational Decision-Making', *Gender, Work and Organisation*, 4(2), April.

—— (1998) 'Models of Disability', in *Disability and Rehabilitation*.

Marks, D., Kendall, T. and Dudley, M. (1998) *Training Needs Assessment for the Assessment and Treatment Unit*, Sheffield: Community Health Sheffield.

Marshall, T.H. (1950) *Citizenship and Social Class*, Cambridge: Cambridge University Press.

Mason, M. (1992) 'Internalised Oppression', in R. Rieser and M. Mason (eds), *Disability Equality in the Classroom: A Human Rights Issue*, London: Disability Equality in Education.

—— (1995) 'The Breaking of Relationships', *Present Time*, January.

Menzies Lyth, I. (1990) 'Social Systems as a Defence Against Anxiety: An Empirical Study of the Nursing Service of a General Hospital', in E. Trist and H. Murray (eds) *The Social Engagement of Social Science*, vol. 1, *The Social-Psychological Perspective*, London: Free Association Books.

Mercer, K. (1986) 'Racism and Transcultural Psychiatry', in P. Miler and B. Rose (eds) *The Power of Psychiatry*, Cambridge: Polity Press.

Merleau-Ponty, M. (1962) *Phenomenology of Perception*, London: Routledge and Kegan Paul.

Miller, E. and Gwynne G. (1972) *A Life Apart: A Pilot Study of Residential Institutions for the Physically Handicapped and the Young Chronic Sick*, London: Tavistock Publications.

Morris, J. (1991) *Pride Against Prejudice: Transforming Attitudes Towards Disability*, London: The Women's Press.

—— (1993) *Independent Lives: Community Care and Disabled People*, London: The Macmillan Press.

—— (1996) *Encounters with Strangers: Feminism and Disability*, Women's Press, London.

Murphy, R. (1987) *The Body Silent*, London: Dent.

Murphy, R.F., Scheer, J, Murphy, Y. and Mack, R. (1988) 'Physical Disability and Social Liminality: A Study in the Rituals of Adversity', *Social Science and Medicine*, 26(2): 235–42.

Murray, N. and May, A. (1988) 'Painful Crisis in Sickle Cell Disease – Patient Perspectives', *British Medical Journal*, 297: 452–54.

Napolitano, S. (1996) 'Mobility Impairment', in G. Hales (ed.) *Beyond Disability*.

Norden, M.F. (1994) *The Cinema of Isolation: A History of Physical Disability in the Movies*, New Brunswick: Rutgers.

—— (1995) 'Politics, Movies and Physical Disability', *Kaleidoscope*, 30, Winter/Spring: 14.

Obholzer, A. and Roberts, Z. (1994) *The Unconscious at Work: Individual and Organisational Stress in the Human Services*, London: Routledge.

Oliver, M. (1990) *The Politics of Disablement*, Basingstoke: Macmillan.

—— (1991) (ed.) *Social Work: Disabled People and Disabling Environments*, London: Jessica Kingsley.

—— (1996) *Understanding Disability: From Theory to Practice*, London: Macmillan.

Oliver, S. (1995) 'Annotation: Self-Injurious Behaviour in Children with Learning Disabilities: Recent Advances in Assessment and Intervention', *Journal of Child Psychology and Psychiatry*, 36: 909–27.

Orbach, S. (1990) 'Gender and Dependency in Psychotherapy', *Journal of Social Work Practice*, 4(314), November: 1–15.

Padden, C. and Humphries, T. (1988) *Deaf in America: Voices from a Culture*, Cambridge, MA: Harvard University Press.

Parker, I. (1998) (ed.) *Social Constructionism, Discourse and Realism*, London: Sage.

Parker, I., Georgaca, E., Harper, D., Mclaughlin, T. and Stowell-Smith, M. (1995) *Deconstructing Psychopathology*, London: Sage.

Parsons, T. (1939) 'The Professions and the Social Structure', *Social Forces*, 17: 457–67.

—— (1951) *The Social System*, London: Routledge and Kegan Paul.

Parsons, T. and Fox, R. (1952) 'Illness, Therapy and the Modern American Family', *Journal of Social Issues*, 8: 31–44.

Partridge, J. (1990) *Changing Faces: The Challenge of Facial Disfigurement*, London: Penguin.

Patterson, K. (1998) 'Disability Studies and Phenomenology: Finding a Space for Both the Carnal and the Political', paper presented at the *Annual British Sociological Association Conference*, Edinburgh.

Patterson, K. and Hughes, B. (1997) 'The Social Model of Disability and the Disappearing Body: Towards a Sociology of Impairment', *Disability and Society*, 12(3), June: 325–40.

Pence, G.E. (1995) *Classical Cases in Medical Ethics: Accounts of Cases That Have Shaped Medical Ethics and Philosophical, Legal and Historical Backgrounds*, New York: McGraw-Hill.

Perry, B., Pollard, R., Blakeley, T., Baker, W. and Vigilante, D. (1995) 'Childhood Trauma, the Neurobiology of Adaptation and "Use-Dependent" Development of the Brain: How "States" Become "Traits" ', *Infant Mental Health Journal*, 16: 271–91.

Pinder, R. (1996) 'Sick-but-fit or Fit-but-sick? Ambiguity and Identity at the Workplace', in C. Barnes and G. Mercer (eds) *Exploring the Divide*.

Piontelli, A. (1992) *From Foetus to Child: An Observational and Psychoanalytic Study*, London: Routledge in association with the Institute of Psycho-Analysis.

Pomerantz, A. (1986) 'Extreme Case Formulations: A New Way of Legitimating Claims', in G. Button, P. Drew and J. Heritage (eds) *Human Studies*, Interaction and Language Use Special Issues, 9L: 219–30.

Pope, A.M. and Tarlov, A.R. (eds) (1991) *Disability in America: Toward a National Agenda for Prevention*, Washington DC: National Academy Press.

Potter, J. and Weatherell, M. (1987) *Discourse and Social Psychology*, London: Sage.

PPR Newsletter (Psychology, Politics, Resistance) (1998) Manchester: Department of Psychology and Speech Pathology, Manchester Metropolitan University.

Pringle, R. (1989) 'Bureaucracies, Rationality and Sexuality: the Case of Secretaries', in J. Hearn, D. Sheppard, P. Tancred-Shefir and G. Burrell, *The Sexuality of Organisation*, London: Sage.

Procter, R. (1988) *Racial Hygiene: Medicine and the Nazis*, Cambridge: Harvard University Press.

Pukulski, J. (1996) 'Cultural Citizenship', *Cultural Studies*, 1(1): 73–86.

Raynor, E. (1991) *The Independent Mind in British Psychoanalysis*, London: Free Association Books.

Richards, B. (1994) *Disciplines of Delight: The Psychoanalysis of Popular Culture*, London: Free Association Books.

Richardson, D. (1996) *Theorising Heterosexuality*, Milton Keynes: Open University Press.

Robertson, J. and Robertson, J. (1989) *Separation and the Very Young*, London: Free Association Books.

Rose, J. (1996) *Freak Like Me*, London: Indigo Press.

Rose, N. (1985)*The Psychological Complex*, London: Routledge and Kegan Paul.

—— (1989) *Governing the Soul: The Shaping of the Private Self*, London: Routledge.

Rose, S., Kamin, J. and Lewontin, R.C. (1984) *Not in Our Genes: Biology, Ideology and Human Nature*, Harmonsworth, Penguin.

Russo, M. (1995) *The Female Grotesque: Risk, Excess and Modernity*, London: Routledge.

Rustin, M. (1992) *The Good Society and the Inner World*, London: Verso.

Ryan, J. with Thomas, F. (1987) *The Politics of Mental Handicap*, London: Free Association Books.

Ryecroft, C. (1972) *A Critical Dictionary of Psychoanalysis*, London: Penguin.

Sacks, O. (1987) *The Man Who Mistook his Wife for a Hat and Other Clinical Tales*, New York: Harper Collins.

Said, E.W. (1995) 'Orientalism', in B. Ashcroft, G. Griffith, H. Tiffin (eds) *The Post-Colonial Studies Reader*, London: Routledge.

Sandhal, C. (1991) 'Performing Disability: Performing Gender: Mark Medoff's Children of a Lesser God and Joan Schenkar's Signs of Life', unpublished thesis submitted in partial fulfilment of the Master of Arts, University of Wisconsin-Madison.

Sandler, J., Holder, A., Dare, C. and Dreher, A. (1997) *Freud's Models of the Mind*, Psychoanalytic Monograph no. 1, London: Karnac Books.

Saxton, M. and Howe, F. (eds) (1988) *With Wings: An Anthology of Literature By and About Women with Disabilities*, London: Virago.

Schlapobersky, J. (1991) 'Editor's Introduction', in R. *Institutes and How to Survive Them: Mental Health Training and Consultation*, London: Routledge.

Schore, A. (1996) 'The Experience-dependent Maturation of a Regulatory System in the Orbital Prefrontal Cortex and the Origin of Developmental

Psychopathology', *Development and Psychopathology*, Cambridge: Cambridge University Press, 59–87.

—— (1998) *Affect Regulation and the Self*, New York: Lawrence Earlbaum.

Scope (1995) 'Talking About Disability Bookmark', London: Scope.

Scott, R.A. (1979) *The Making of Blind Men: A Study of Adult Socialization*, New York: Russell Sage Foundation.

Scull, A.(1993) *The Most Solitary of Afflictions: Madness and Society in Britain, 1700–1900*, New Haven, CT: Yale University Press.

Shaban, N. (1996) 'Supercrips and Normals', for *Without Walls* series, Fulcrum Productions Limited, for Channel 4, March.

Shakespeare, T. (1994) 'Cultural Representation of Disabled People: Dustbins for Disavowal?', *Disability and Society*, 9(3).

—— (1998) *The Disability Studies Reader: Social Science Perspective*, London: Cassell.

Shakespeare, T., Gillespie-Sells, K. and Davies, D. (1996) *The Sexual Politics of Disability*, London: Cassell.

Shapiro, E.R. and Carr, A.W. (1991) *Lost in Familiar Places: Creating New Connections Between the Individual and Society*, New Haven, CT: Yale University Press.

Shapiro, J.P. (1994) *No Pity: People with Disabilities Forging a New Civil Rights Movement*, New York: Times Books.

Shearer, A. (1996) 'Think Positive! Advice on Presenting People with Mental Handicap', in P. Mittler with V. Sinason (eds) *Changing Policy and Practice for People with Learning Disabilities*, London: Cassell Educational, pp. 205–18.

Shildrick, M. (1996) *Leaky Bodies and Boundaries: Feminism, Postmodernism and (Bio)Ethics*, London: Routledge.

Shilling, C. (1993) *The Body and Social Theory*, London: Sage.

—— (1997) 'The Body and Difference', in K. Woodward (ed.) *Identity and Difference*, London: Sage.

Sibley, D. (1996) *Geographies of Exclusion*, London: Routledge.

Sinason, V. (1992) *Mental Handicap and the Human Condition*, London: Free Association Books.

—— (1997) 'Gender-Linked Issues in Psychotherapy with Abused and Learning Disabled Female Patients', in J. Raphael-Leff and R. Jozef Perelberg (eds) *Female Experience: Three Generations of British Women Psychoanalysts on Work With Women*, London: Routledge.

—— (1998) personal communication in the Mental Handicap Workshop at the Tavistock Clinic.

Sivanandan, A. (1983) 'Rat and the Degradation of Black Struggle', *Race and Class*, 24(2): 1–33.

Skynner, R. (1991) *Institutes and How to Survive Them: Mental Health Training and Consultation*, London: Routledge.

Slater, D. (1998) 'Needs/Wants', in C. Jenks (ed.) *Core Sociological Dichotomies*.

Sobsey, R. (1994) *Violence and Abuse in the Lives of People With Disabilities*, London: Brookes.

Solity, J. (1992) *Special Education*, London: Cassell Educational.

Sontag, S. (1991) 'Illness as Metaphor', in *Illness as Metaphor and Aids and its Metaphors*, New York: Doubleday Anchor.

Stone, D.A. (1985) *The Disabled State*, Basingstoke: Macmillan.

Stone, E. (1996) 'A Law to Protect, a Law to Prevent: Contextualising Disability Legislation in China', *Disability and Society*, 11(4), December.

Swain, J., Finkelstein, V., French, S. and Oliver, M. (1994) *Disabling Barriers – Enabling Environments*, London: Sage in association with the Open University Press.

Swann, W. (ed.) (1986) *The Practice of Special Education*, Oxford: Blackwell and Oxford University Press.

Symington, N. (1986) *The Analytic Experience: Lectures from the Tavistock*, London: Free Association Books.

Teichman, J. (1996) *Social Ethics*, Oxford: Basil Blackwell.

Thomas, F. (1987) 'Everyday Life on the Ward', in J. Ryan with F. Thomas *The Politics of Mental Handicap*, London: Free Association Books.

Tomlinson, S. (1981) *Educational Subnormality: A Study in Decision-Making*, London: Routledge and Kegan Paul.

—— (1982) *A Sociology of Special Education*, London: Routledge and Kegan Paul.

Travarthen, C. and Aitken, K. (1994) 'Brain Development, Infant Communication and Empathy Disorders: Intrinsic Factors in Child Mental Health, *Development and Psychopathology*, 6: 597–633.

Tregaskis, C. (1998) 'Life Beyond Paid Employment: Disabled Women's Experiences of Giving Up Work', unpublished dissertation in partial fulfilment of the MA Disability Studies, Centre for Psychotherapeutic Studies, Sheffield University.

Turner, B.S. (1995) *Medical Power and Social Knowledge*, London: Sage.

Tustin, F. (1992) *Autistic States in Childhood*, revised edn, London: Routledge.

Van der Kolk, B. and Greenberg, M. (1987) 'The Psychobiology of the Trauma Response: Hyperarousal, Constriction and Addiction to Traumatic Reexposure', *Psychological Trauma*, pp. 63–87.

Van Rooyan, J. (1997) 'There's No Such Thing As A Building', *NewSquiggle: The Newsletter of the Squiggle Foundation*, 1, Autumn: 5–6

Walker, D. (1998) 'Jobs for Life', *The Guardian*, 24 November: 17.

Walmsley, B. (1997) 'A Textual Analysis of the Representation of Disability in "The Walk": An Episode of the X-Files', unpublished dissertation in partial fulfilment of the MA Disability Studies, Centre for Psychotherapeutic Studies, Sheffield University.

Walmsley, J. (1994) ' "Talking to Top People": Some Issues Relating to the Citizenship of People With Learning Difficulties', in J. Swain *et al.* (eds) *Disabling Barriers.*

Weisman, L. (1992) *Discrimination By Design*, Champaign, IL: University of Illinois Press.

Wendell, S. (1996) *The Rejected Body*, London: Routledge.

Wilkinson, S. and Kitzinger, S. (eds) *Representing the Other: A Feminism and Psychology Reader*, London: Sage.

Williams, C. (1995) *Invisible Victims: Crime and Abuse Against People With Learning Difficulties*, London: Jessica Kingsley.

Williams, D. (1994) *Nobody Nowhere: the Extraordinary Autobiography of An Autistic*, New York: Avon Books.

Williams, G. (1984) 'The Genesis of Chronic Illness: Narrative Reconstruction', *Sociology of Health and Illness*, 6: 175–200.

Williamson, J. (1997) 'Survival of the Thinnest', *The Guardian, Weekend* section, 22 March.

Winnicott, D.W. (1960) 'The Theory of Parent Infant Relationship', *International Journal of Psychoanalysis*, 41(585): 37–55.

—— (1963) 'Fear of Breakdown', in D.W. Winnicott, R. Shepherd and M. Davis (eds) (1989) *Psycho-Analytic Explorations*, London: Karnac.

—— (1971) 'Mirror-Role of Mother and Family in Child Development', *Playing and Reality*, London: Tavistock.

—— (1992a) *Through Paediatrics to Psycho-Analysis*, London: Karnac Books and the Institute of Psycho-Analysis.

—— (1992b [1954]) 'Anxiety Associated with Insecurity, in *Through Paediatrics to Psycho-Analysis.*

Wolfenberger, W. (1994) 'Lets Hang Up "Quality of Life" as a Hopeless Term', in D. Goode (ed.) *Quality of Life for Persons with Disabilities: International Perspectives and Issues*, Cambridge, MA: Brookline Books.

Wolfenstein, E.V. (1993) *Psychoanalytic Marxism: Groundwork*, London: Free Association Books.

Wood, P. (1981) *International Classification of Impairments, Disabilities and Handicaps*, Geneva: World Health Organisation.

Woodhead, M. (1990) 'Psychology and the Cultural Construction of Children's Needs', in A. James and A. Prout (eds) *Constructing and Reconstructing Childhood: Contemporary Issues in the Sociological Study of Childhood*, London: The Falmer Press.

Wright, K. (1991) *Vision and Separation: Between Mother and Baby*, London: Free Association Books.

Young, I.M. (1989) 'Polity and Group Difference: A Critique of the Idea of Universal Citizenship', *Ethics*, 99: 250–74.

Young, R.M. (1970) *Mind, Brain and Adaptation*, Oxford: Clarendon Press.

Zola, I.K. (ed.) (1982) *Ordinary Lives: Voices of Disability and Disease*, Cambridge, MA: Applewood Books.

—— (1985) 'Depictions of Disability: Metaphor, Message and Medium in the Media: A Research and Political Agenda', *The Social Science Journal*, 22(4), 5–17.

—— (1988) 'Ageing and Disability: Towards a Unifying Agenda', *Educational Gerontology*, 14: 365–87.

Index

Note: The letter n following a page number indicates a reference in the notes.